ROSY REYNOLDS PhD graduated from Cambridge University in 1978 and was a bio-medical researcher at University College London for several years. She is an experienced teacher and writer whose work involves people in all aspects of medicine, the patients as well as the professionals. Her recently published work includes *Bladder Problems: A Complete Self-Help Guide* (Thorsons 1991).

Overcoming Common Problems Series

For a full list of titles please contact
Sheldon Press, Marylebone Road, London NW1 4DU

Beating the Blues
SUSAN TANNER AND JILLIAN
BALL

Birth Over Thirty
SHEILA KITZINGER

Body Language
How to read others' thoughts by their
gestures
ALLAN PEASE

Calm Down
How to cope with frustration and anger
DR PAUL HAUCK

Changing Course
How to take charge of your career
SUE DYSON AND STEPHEN HOARE

Comfort for Depression
JANET HORWOOD

Complete Public Speaker
GYLES BRANDRETH

Coping Successfully with Migraine
SUE DYSON

**Coping Successfully with Your Child's
Asthma**
DR PAUL CARSON

**Coping Successfully with Your Hyperactive
Child**
DR PAUL CARSON

**Coping Successfully with Your Irritable
Bowel**
ROSEMARY NICOL

**Coping Successfully with Your Second
Child**
FIONA MARSHALL

Coping with Anxiety and Depression
SHIRLEY TRICKETT

Coping with Blushing
DR ROBERT EDELMANN

Coping with Cot Death
SARAH MURPHY

Coping with Depression and Elation
DR PATRICK McKEON

Coping with Stress
DR GEORGIA WITKIN-LANOIL

Coping with Strokes
DR TOM SMITH

Coping with Suicide
DR DONALD SCOTT

Coping with Thrush
CAROLINE CLAYTON

Curing Arthritis – The Drug-Free Way
MARGARET HILLS

Curing Arthritis Diet Book
MARGARET HILLS

**Curing Coughs, Colds and Flu – The
Drug-Free Way**
MARGARET HILLS

Curing Illness – The Drug-Free Way
MARGARET HILLS

Depression
DR PAUL HAUCK

Divorce and Separation
ANGELA WILLANS

Don't Blame Me!
How to stop blaming yourself
and other people
TONY GOUGH

**Everything You Need to Know about
Adoption**
MAGGIE JONES

**Everything You Need to Know about
Osteoporosis**
ROSEMARY NICOL

**Everything You Need to Know about
Shingles**
DR ROBERT YOUNGSON

**Family First Aid and Emergency
Handbook**
DR ANDREW STANWAY

Feverfew
DR STEWART JOHNSON

Overcoming Common Problems Series

Overcoming Common Problems Series

Overcoming Common Problems

COPING SUCCESSFULLY WITH PROSTATE PROBLEMS

Rosy Reynolds

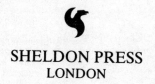

SHELDON PRESS
LONDON

First published in Great Britain
Sheldon Press, SPCK, Marylebone Road, London NW1 4DU

British Library Cataloguing-in-Publication Data
A catalogue record for this book is available from the British Library
ISBN 0–85969–659–6

Photoset by Deltatype Ltd, Ellesmere Port, Cheshire
Printed in Great Britain by Biddles Ltd, Guildford and King's Lynn

For my parents

Contents

Acknowledgements

With thanks to: Marian Budd SRN SCM, P. J. Burney MBChB MRCGP, Trevor Coleman, Henry Dixon, Nick Dixon PhD BM BCh, R. C. L. Feneley MA MChir FRCS, Rachel M. Gunary MA MSc CClinPsych, Tony Hinchliffe, Wendy Hurn SRN SCM, Lyn Kirkwood RGN, Mike Lewis MRCGP MB BS, A. H. Mayor BSc MB BS MRCP FCAnaes, Dr James Mulvein FCAnaes, Jim Panting, Derek Rogers and Corinne Wong SRN SCM, who so much enlivened my researches.

1

Introduction

The prostate gland is notorious for the trouble it causes to older men. Hundreds of thousands of men suffer – with sleep disturbed by the need to get up to empty their bladders several times a night, social activities curtailed by the need always to be in easy reach of a toilet, a feeble unsatisfying flow of urine and sometimes even a complete and painful inability to pass urine at all – all because of a benign enlargement of the prostate gland.

As a result, over 40,000 operations to remove the prostate (prostatectomies) are done each year in Britain. In America, where prostate removal ranks in the top four of operations on men (rivalled only by cataract removal, hernia repair and operations on the gall bladder), nearly 400,000 prostatectomies are performed at an estimated cost of over $4,000 each (a total of over 1,500 million dollars). What is it about this gland, no larger than a chestnut in a healthy state, which makes it so liable to cause trouble?

The prostate encircles the tube which carries urine out of the bladder, like an armband around a young swimmer's arm or the cuff used to measure blood pressure. When it enlarges it presses on the pipe, just as the inflated band or cuff presses on the arm, and blocks the flow of urine either partially or completely. The result is a hesitant start to urination and a slow flow. Later, the bladder is often unable to empty completely and more annoying symptoms develop such as needing to pee frequently and urgently, day and night.

As to why the gland enlarges in the first place, researchers are not so sure, although it is very probably related to the fact that prostate growth depends on the male hormone testosterone. Those organs which depend on sex hormones do seem to be particularly prone to disorders of growth, both benign and malignant. Women commonly suffer from benign growths in the breasts and womb (and a third of all female cancers occur in these organs) while men commonly suffer benign enlargement of the prostate (and one tenth of all male cancers occur here).

Whatever the exact cause of a man's benign prostate enlargement, it begins a long time before any symptoms become noticeable, probably forty years or more before. At some time in his

1

twenties, when other young men's prostates stop growing, his continues to enlarge. Growing very, very slowly, but steadily and insidiously, it may take years before it even begins to constrict the outflow pipe, and the slowing may happen so gradually that it is several years more before it is noticed. Once the constriction is severe enough to cause noticeable symptoms, any further growth in the gland is likely to make them worse. If the process continues, there is a possibility of irreversible damage to the bladder and, crucially, to the kidneys.

Who develops prostate enlargement? The answer is anyone and everyone – anyone in the sense that we do not know of anything which increases or decreases the risk of the disease, so we cannot predict who is most likely to suffer, and everyone in the sense that by the age of 85, 90 per cent of men have microscopic signs of the changes in the prostate which lead to enlargement, and workers believe that practically all men would show these changes if they lived long enough.

Prostate enlargement becomes very much commoner with increasing age. At 35, less than ten per cent of men have even microscopic signs of it but by 75 about 80 per cent have microscopic changes in the prostate tissue. Roughly speaking, at all ages, half of those with microscopic changes have a detectable enlargement of the gland and half of those with actual enlargement have notable symptoms because of it. Therefore, roughly a fifth of men aged 75 have urinary symptoms due to prostate enlargement. A larger proportion of men than this have some bladder problems, though, because there are other causes apart from prostate enlargement. About a third of men over the age of 60 have several symptoms such as needing to pee very frequently or very urgently in the day, or having to get up twice or more at night.

In British practice, the rough 'rule of halves' applies to the proportion of men having surgery, so by the age of 80 approximately one man in ten will have had a prostatectomy to remove the troublesome gland. Most operations are done between 65 and 85 but it is a mistake to think that you are immune if you are younger than this. Prostatectomy is very rare under the age of 45, but a fifth of all the operations are for men between 45 and 65. This corresponds to about one man in six hundred of that age having the operation each year. Between 65 and 75, roughly one man in a hundred has a prostatectomy each year, and one in seventy each year between the ages of 75 and 85.

The proportion of men having surgery varies enormously from country to country. Even within a country, and after correcting for the numbers of men of different ages, operations are done two and a half times more frequently in some areas than others. In the USA, men are at least twice as likely to have a prostatectomy as men in Britain, perhaps as much as three times as likely. In fact, the operation has been targeted by American 'second opinion programs' as one that should be reduced in number as it is thought to be being performed unnecessarily in some cases.

Far fewer men seek medical help than have symptoms, most probably because they see their diffiulties as an inevitable aspect of ageing. Many physical abilities decline with age, and it has been known for centuries that the urinary torrent of youth is likely to diminish to a sad trickle in later years. Since ageing is unavoidable, many men accept their failing urination as unavoidable too.

While such stoicism would be commendable in the face of a truly insoluble problem, it is neither necessary nor wise in this case. Until your symptoms are properly investigated, you do not know their cause. Usually, in older men, it is benign enlargement of the prostate gland but there are other possibilities (see Chapter 3) which it would be important to detect and treat. Even where the symptoms are caused by straightforward enlargement, they are likely to worsen and there is a risk of damage to your kidneys. Now that treatment is effective and available, it makes sense to seek it while you are in fair health and before the progression of the disease turns you into a high-risk emergency case.

This book should help you whether you are already on a waiting list for surgery or have just noticed some symptoms and are wondering whether you should consult a doctor. It is in three parts: understanding your illness and its symptoms, investigating it and choosing treatment, and having the typical operation.

The first part (Chapters 2 and 3) is of general interest. Chapter 2 describes the symptoms you may have and how common they are. Chapter 3 explains how the system works and how an enlarged prostate causes the trouble it does; it also covers other conditions which can cause similar symptoms.

The second part (Chapters 4 and 5) is to help you to understand the factors to be considered in choosing a particular treatment. Chapter 4 describes the medical tests that may be done and what you can learn from them, starting with simple checks you can do yourself and going on to your first visit to your family doctor and possible sophisticated hospital tests. Chapter 5 contains details of various treatments available and their advantages and disadvantages so that, if you choose to, you will be in a position to participate fully in the decision about how best to tackle the problem.

The third part (Chapters 6, 7 and 8) is a practical guide to surgical treatment, including the possible wait for an operation. Chapter 6 has advice on living with the problem until it is treated. Chapter 7 describes the hospital stay for a prostate operation in detail, and Chapter 8 tells you what to expect and what to do to promote your own recovery when you return home.

A note about technical terms

Medical terms are a handy shorthand to healthcare professionals but most of them are unnecessary for the rest of us. I explain quite a few in this book, to help you understand what the doctors and nurses may be saying, but I have tried to avoid using them unnecessarily. Those that I do use, and a few more, are included in the glossary (page 119) for easy reference.

There are just a few technical terms which I cannot avoid using repeatedly, and the most unavoidable of all (after prostate) is *urethra*. This is the name of the tube which carries urine from the bladder to the outside, passing through the prostate and the penis on its way. It goes, literally, to the core of the problem and there is no way to describe the problem or the treatment without mentioning it often.

One term which I do avoid throughout the book, because it is such a complicated mouthful, is the correct medical name for the prostate enlargement itself. The kind of prostate enlargement which most men get, the kind which this book is mainly about and which I usually refer to simply as 'prostate enlargement', is correctly called *benign prostatic hyperplasia* (BPH, also sometimes called benign prostatic *hypertrophy*). Hyperplasia means that the enlargement is brought about by the growth of new cells. Benign, in this context, means that the new prostatic growth has no tendency to spread or seed itself into other parts of the body, i.e. it is not malignant. It does not mean harmless. So-called 'benign' prostatic hyperplasia can continue for years causing nothing more than annoyance but equally, left untreated, it can cause severe harm. You should take medical advice. The rest of the book explains why in more detail, and where that advice may lead.

2
Symptoms

It is useful to know what symptoms can appear in your urinary system, and what names the doctors use for them. It helps you to recognize your problem and to describe it more precisely, and it is interesting to know a little about what the symptoms may mean. However, it is not wise to try to do your own diagnosis and decide on that basis whether or not you should see a doctor. Apart from getting up a few times at night for a pee, or having minor dribbles shortly after you finish peeing, any other changes in your urinary habits which are big enough to notice are big enough to consult a doctor about.

Benign prostatic enlargement is not the only possible cause of urinary symptoms (see Chapter 3) and it is worth finding out the exact cause, discovering whether it is trivial or serious, and treating it, if appropriate, before it progresses beyond annoyance to real damage. You cannot rely on the symptoms to tell what the underlying disorder is. They have an uncertain connection with the original disease and vary from case to case, so it takes more detailed tests (Chapter 4) to identify the root cause of the problem for sure.

Obstructive symptoms

The so-called obstructive symptoms do not prove that there is an obstruction to the flow of urine, although they are the sort of symptoms that you would logically expect from obstruction and they are present in about three-quarters of men having operations for prostate enlargement. They might equally logically be caused by weakness in the bladder muscle, or by a failure of coordination between the muscles with the job of expelling urine and those with the job of retaining it.

Hesitancy

Hesitancy means difficulty in getting the flow of urine started, so that instead of waiting a few seconds before starting to pee you might have to wait a minute or more. It seems as if the bladder muscle has difficulty in contracting forcefully enough to open the urethra. Some younger men, who pee quite normally at home, have

5

extreme difficulty in doing so in public: psychological factors such as embarrassment and self-consciousness play a part here and the difficulty has been dubbed 'anxious bladder' although of course it is not the bladder who is anxious.

Poor stream

Poor stream is meant to refer to a slow flow of urine at the toilet. Like a quarter of all men over sixty, you may notice it is as a thin stream, or as an inability to pee as high or as far as you used to, or as a prolonged time of urinating. If you are always emptying very small volumes of urine, the flow will appear slow whether or not there is an obstruction because it will hardly have time to get started before it has to stop again.

The urine stream may also change shape, splitting into two or spraying. This is not typical of prostate enlargement but do mention it when you describe your symptoms to your doctor. It may indicate a constriction nearer the tip of the penis.

Intermittent flow

Intermittent flow is a more severe form of poor stream. The flow comes in fits and starts because the bladder muscle cannot maintain the pressure needed to hold the urethra open throughout urination.

Terminal dribble, post-micturition dribble

Intermittent flow is particularly likely towards the end of urination when the bladder muscle begins to relax again and the pressure on the urine falls. The urethra tends to close or partly close before the bladder has quite finished emptying and, typically, the last part of the urine is emptied in a series of unsatisfying dribbles. This is terminal dribble.

Post-micturition dribble (after-dribble) is not the same thing as terminal dribble. With after-dribble, a small amount of urine escapes several seconds after the end of urination. This has less to do with obstruction and more to do with the strength and coordination of the muscles in and around the urethra. It does not usually signify anything particular, and a method to prevent the dribble wetting your underwear or trousers is given in Chapter 6, (see page 74).

Up to a quarter of men over sixty have occasional unwanted dribbles of urine but the surveys have not distinguished between dribbles which happen after urination and those which happen before, when it has been impossible to reach a toilet quickly enough.

Feeling of incomplete emptying

This is exactly what is says: you feel that there is urine left in your bladder even though you have just finished peeing, and you may well be right. The bladder muscle may not be able to overcome the obstruction effectively enough to empty itself completely. You can also suffer from a feeling that you need to empty your bladder again when in fact it is empty. This often happens with urinary infections and with stones in the bladder.

Retention

Retention is less common than the other obstructive symptoms with around one in ten men having chronic retention when they go for prostate surgery, and one in three having had an attack of acute retention.

Chronic retention

If your bladder does not empty itself completely, it will contain some residual urine after using the toilet. If there is a large volume of residual urine, half a pint (300 ml) or so, the doctors start to call this a chronic retention of urine rather than a residual volume. 'Chronic' means that the situation is longstanding; it does not say anything about its seriousness. Chronic retention is painless so you may not realize that you have it although you may notice the swelling of your lower abdomen over the full bladder, or find that you need to let your belt out a notch or two.

Acute retention

Acute retention, on the other hand, is sudden and painful. You are completely unable to pee although your bladder feels as if it has reached bursting point. You may find that you can relieve yourself when lying in a warm bath but, if not, do not delay in seeking medical help.

Acute retention strikes unpredictably. Sometimes it is the first unmistakeable sign of prostate enlargement, sometimes it follows on from chronic retention, and sometimes it has nothing to do with the prostate whatsoever. Acute retention can be brought on in people with no previous urinary problems, for example by drugs given to relieve heart failure, or following an operation.

Irritative symptoms

As with the obstructive symptoms which do not prove the existence of obstruction, the so-called irritative symptoms do not prove the existence of irritation and certainly do not prove the existence of a prostate problem. Men needing treatment for prostate enlargement are twice as likely to have these symptoms as other men of the same age, but many men with irritative symptoms have no prostate trouble. Other possible causes include urinary infection and bladder instability (see Chapter 3, pages 26 and 27).

Frequency

Frequency is a common symptom, affecting about a third of men over 60. It means urinating unusually often, which is usually taken to be seven or more times in the waking day. Most people pee between four and six times a day, and can last quite comfortably for four hours between visits to the toilet. One trivial cause of frequency is drinking too much, out of habit. If you have a cup of tea every hour, then naturally you will need to empty your bladder every couple of hours; it does not mean that there is anything wrong with you. However, you should certainly consult a doctor if you are drinking that much because you are really that thirsty. More typically, a man who has frequency pees very small amounts each time although he drinks normally and produces a normal volume of urine over the day.

Urgency, urge incontinence

Urgency is an urgent feeling of wanting to empty your bladder, or a feeling of impending emptying irrespective of wanting. Urge incontinence is the resulting unwanted loss of urine if you cannot hold out against the urgency for long enough to reach a toilet and undo your clothing. The older you are, the more likely you are to have urgency. It affects about a quarter of men in their sixties and over a third of men between 70 and 85.

Nocturia

Nocturia means waking and needing to empty your bladder during the night. It is often simply a continuation of daytime frequency but it can occur on its own. In that case, the fault probably lies not with your bladder but with your kidneys producing more urine than normal at night. This may happen if you have a sedentary lifestyle which allows fluid to pool in your legs during the day. This excess fluid has to be excreted when it returns to the bloodstream while you are lying down at night.

Nocturia is not at all uncommon in older people with a quarter of men over 60 visiting the toilet twice or more each night. A doctor may consider it more or less par for the course if you have to get up once a night at the age of 65, twice at 75 and three times at 85. He is unlikely to worry unless the trips are more frequent than this, or there are other symptoms as well.

Other symptoms

Incontinence

There are various forms of incontinence in addition to the urge incontinence mentioned above. Bedwetting is one, and losing urine soon after you fall asleep can happen when you have a chronic retention of urine. Chronic retention can also go on to cause continuous dribbling incontinence when the pressure in the bladder is raised so much that urine is squeezed out constantly. In stress incontinence, urine is lost in spurts as a result of physical stresses such as coughing or stumbling; it is unusual in men except shortly after prostate surgery or following pelvic injuries.

Estimates for how widespread a problem incontinence is vary according to the definition used. Minor dribbles, which are about ten times more common than major problems, affect up to a quarter of men over 60.

Incontinence is not an inevitable part of old age; it is a symptom of something wrong. Often the cause can be treated. Even if it cannot, there are all sorts of aids now available to help you manage incontinence with the minimum of embarrassment and social inconvenience. Seek help. If you are too embarrassed to talk to your doctor, think about talking to a different doctor, or the practice or district nurse, or the community continence adviser. Continence advisers are specialist nurses who deal with bladder control problems the whole time; the ones I have met are immensely approachable and almost impossible to embarrass. You can find out whether a continence adviser works in your area by asking in your doctor's surgery or by phoning the local hospital or community health council.

Haematuria

Haematuria means blood in the urine. There are all sorts of causes for this, some fairly innocuous, others not, so it is essential to see a doctor within a day or two even if the bleeding seems to have stopped.

Haemospermia

This means blood in the semen. Unless there are other symptoms as well, it is most unlikely to indicate anything seriously wrong but it is wise to take medical advice.

Pain (dysuria, strangury)

Pain when you pee is called 'dysuria'. It is useful to notice what sort of pain it is, and where it is. Urinary infections, for example, tend to give a stinging or burning pain along the whole length of the penis. Strangury is a cramp-like pain, mainly in the bladder area itself, which feels as if it would go away if only you could pee freely, but the urine actually comes out drop by drop or not at all. Stones in the bladder can cause strangury because the bladder tries to eject them just as it would eject a full load of urine, but however hard it contracts the stones remain in place.

Haemorrhoids (piles)

Haemorrhoids are not exactly a symptom of prostate enlargement but they may well be worse if an enlarged prostate is putting pressure on nearby blood vessels. If yours are playing you up, and you know that you have a prostate problem too, take comfort in the hope that a prostate operation will ease both problems at once.

Other symptoms

A symptom like being tired all the time has many possible causes. It may be a physical result of prostate enlargement, with kidney damage causing anaemia (unusual) or with losing sleep from having to get up to pee so often (common). It may be a psychological result, with depression triggered off by being fed up with the urinary symptoms. It may have nothing to do with your prostate; you may have some other illness, or simply be working too hard, or worrying over something and losing sleep because of that. However, the fact that tiredness is a non-specific symptom does not make it an insignificant one. It is a clue and it needs to be considered along with all the other clues.

The same goes for other symptoms such as losing your appetite, being thirstier than usual or having pains in other parts of the body. Mention them all to your doctor.

3

How the System Works
and What Goes Wrong

The normal working of the system

Layout

The urinary system starts with the kidneys. These are packed in fat and firmly attached to the back just below the lower ribs. They filter the blood, retaining the useful substances and producing urine containing the waste products, so they have a very rich blood supply. Each one has a tube called a ureter (not to be confused with the urethra) which carries the urine down to the bladder (see Figure 1).

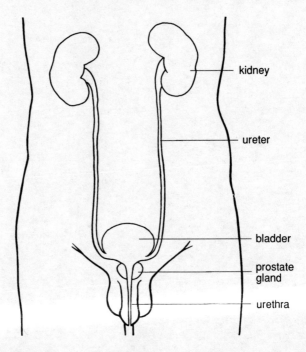

Fig. 1 Schematic view from the front to show the main parts of the urinary system, and the prostate gland.

The bladder is a muscular bag that stores the urine until a suitable time for releasing it. It lies low in the abdomen at about the level of the pubic bone, the bone you can feel under your pubic hair. Urine leaves the bladder through a single tube called the urethra.

The bladder and the top part of the urethra are supported by pairs of large muscles called the pelvic floor muscles which are slung across the pelvis from front to back. These are joined in the middle for most of their length, with small gaps to allow the urethra and the anal canal to run through and reach the outside. The urethra runs from the base of the bladder, through the pelvic floor, forwards to the base of the penis and down to the outside at the tip of the penis (see Figure 2).

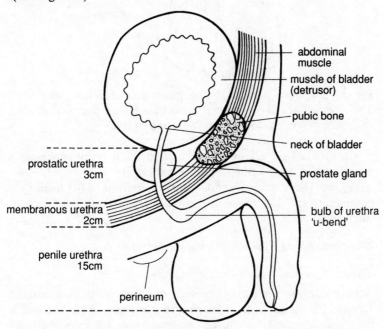

abdominal muscle

muscle of bladder (detrusor)

pubic bone

neck of bladder

prostate gland

bulb of urethra 'u-bend'

prostatic urethra 3cm

membranous urethra 2cm

penile urethra 15cm

perineum

Fig. 2 The lower urinary system and prostate gland seen from the right side, showing the support given by the pelvic floor and the lengths of the three sections of the urethra.

The urethra has a sexual function as well as a urinary function. The sperm which is produced in the testicles and matured in the epididymes is carried through the sperm ducts in a long loop up to the top end of the urethra. Other glands – notably the prostate gland and the seminal vesicles – add secretions to the sperm along the way and the resulting mixture, semen, reaches the outside along the urethra (see Figure 3).

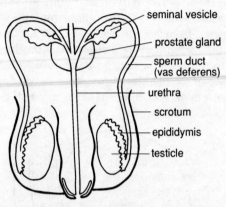

seminal vesicle

prostate gland

sperm duct
(vas deferens)

urethra

scrotum

epididymis

testicle

Fig. 3 The main parts of the genital system seen from the front. The testicles are drawn further apart than in real life, as if the left and right halves of the scrotum were separate sacs.

The prostate gland is at the spaghetti junction of this system. It is a small gland, around the size of a chestnut, just below the bladder neck, just above the pelvic floor and just in front of the rectum. It completely encircles the urethra at the point where the two sperm ducts join.

Urine production – the workings of the kidneys

The need for removal of waste chemicals

A healthy body is in a very fine state of chemical balance, and the kidneys play a key role in keeping that balance. Even the useful substances in food have to be converted into others as the body makes use of them for energy or for replacing cells that have broken down, and the conversion process inevitably produces chemical by-products and wastes. Other substances in the diet may be useless or even toxic and these obviously have to be removed, either directly or after being converted to less harmful substances. In addition, some substances in the diet are used unchanged in the body, salt and water for example, but their amounts must be carefully controlled by excreting any excess.

14

Apart from varying amounts of salt and water, the main waste products in urine are the products of protein breakdown such as urea and creatinine.

Filtration and the need for a pressure difference

The kidneys work, quite literally, by filtering the blood. The filter is so fine that it keeps back the blood cells and the large protein molecules but lets through all the truly soluble substances such as sugars and salts. Then the useful substances are pumped back into the blood in the quantities required – usually all of the sugar, most of the water and most of the salts.

Because the filter is so fine, there needs to be quite a pressure difference to drive the blood through it. This is provided by the blood pressure which is sufficient so long as the urine drains away freely at low pressure. If the flow is prevented and urine backs up to the kidney at high pressure, the blood pressure is not enough to force liquid through the filter and urine production fails.

Control of urine production

Urine production can never be switched off completely. Blood is always entering the kidney, being filtered and producing urine which drains into the bladder. However, the amount of urine you produce is controlled according to the amount of water in your body.

If you are short of water, the pituitary gland in your brain produces a hormone called antidiuretic hormone (ADH). This hormone travels in the bloodstream to the kidneys and makes them pump back as much water as possible from the urine into the blood. The small volume of urine which is produced contains all the usual waste so it is dark yellow and smelly. If you have drunk a great deal, the brain stops producing ADH and the kidneys allow the water to remain in the urine which is then very pale and practically odourless. ADH secretion has a daily rhythm, with more of it produced at night to slow overnight urine production and make night-time bladder emptying unnecessary.

There are also controls that influence your thirst and the movement of salts in the kidneys so that no matter what you eat or drink initially, your body tries to stabilize to the correct volume of water and the correct concentration of salt.

However, the system is not fool-proof. The detectors for water volume and salt concentration are in the central areas of the system

– in the brain and near the heart. If the liquid is held somewhere else, around puffy ankles, for instance, it will not be detected and urine production will not be increased to remove it until it returns to the central circulation. This is just like a thermostat in the hall of a house which does not switch on the central heating for a cold bedroom until the cold spreads to the hall. Also, it takes time for the controls to work. If you have been short of water and start drinking, it will be some time before the urine production speeds up to match your intake, and fast production will continue for some time after you stop drinking.

Other functions of the kidneys

The kidneys also have a role in the control of blood pressure and in the production of red blood cells. Kidney damage affects these aspects too; it tends to lead to high blood pressure and anaemia.

Urine storage

The storage tank (bladder)

The bladder is made of tough and extremely stretchy muscle, the detrusor muscle. It is not really like a balloon because, when it is working properly, it stays relaxed while it fills and stretches very easily so that the pressure inside hardly changes. A typical normal bladder can hold almost a pint (500 ml) when filled to capacity, but there is a lot of variation from one person to another.

The piping and taps (urethra and sphincters)

The urethra which carries the urine from the bladder to the outside is a tube about eight inches (20 cm) long. The tube is formed of muscle and lined with fine skin or epithelium. Different names are given to the different sections of the urethra as shown in Figure 2.

The muscle in the urethral wall is thickest in the membranous urethra, where the urethra is making its way through the pelvic floor muscles. Here, and in the prostatic urethra above, the muscles in and around the urethral wall are responsible for holding the tube closed when urine flow is not required. These rings of muscle are the sphincters which act as taps, controlling the opening and closing of the urethra. Anatomists recognize separate internal and external sphincters, involuntary and voluntary sphincters, sphincters of different types of muscle, but these details overcomplicate the picture for our purposes. The important point is that there is spare capacity in the system. One area of sphincter may be injured, or even surgically removed, but the remaining area is still well able to maintain a leakproof seal (see Figures 4 and 5).

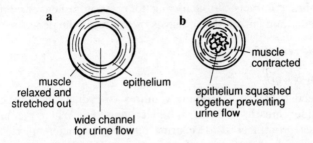

Fig. 4 Cross-sections of the urethra to show how the sphincters work. **a** With the sphincter muscles relaxed the tube can dilate and urine can flow. The epithelium is a fine resilient 'skin' covering the inner surface of the urethra. **b** The sphincter muscles contracted. The muscle fibres are arranged in circles around the urethra so that when they shorten they constrict the tube, the epithelium is squashed into any remaining crevices and urine flow is prevented.

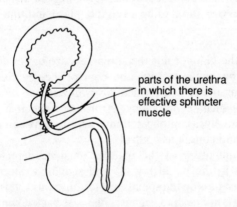

Fig. 5 A side view of the system to show which parts of the urethra have effective sphincter muscle in and around them.

Part of the sphincter mechanism is under direct conscious control and this is the part you activate when you choose to stop the flow of urine suddenly in midstream. It is only possible to hold urine in this way for short periods. Normally, closure is maintained by muscles working 'autonomically', controlled by reflexes involving nerve cells in the spine or in lower parts of the brain.

During sex, the muscle of the bladder neck and upper prostatic urethra contracts automatically to prevent semen entering the bladder and ensure that it leaves the body via the penis.

Urine removal

How it works

Effective bladder emptying requires co-ordination between the bladder muscle and the sphincter muscles. When the bladder muscle contracts to force urine out, the sphincter muscles must relax to allow the urine to flow unhindered. In these circumstances, the bladder will empty completely. Afterwards, the sphincters should contract to close the urethra again and the bladder muscle should relax to allow the bladder to refill at low pressure. Reflex centres in the spinal cord and lower brain are able to organize this coordination and complete emptying does not depend on consciousness.

However, true bladder control does require conscious input from the brain as it involves recognizing the urge to urinate, suppressing it as necessary and finding a suitable place and time.

How it is controlled

Neither the bladder not the sphincters are under direct conscious control, but your decisions do control the muscles indirectly by influencing the reflexes which govern their activities. Full bladder control, which seems almost effortless when it is working well, actually involves complicated interactions between muscles, nerve reflexes and conscious controls.

First, the filling of the bladder must be detected (by stretch detectors in the bladder wall) and signalled (along nerves); the signal must pass up the spinal cord to conscious levels of the brain. If emptying is not desired, signals must pass back down the spinal cord to inhibit the reflexes which would otherwise bring about automatic emptying. When urination is wanted to begin, the inhibition is lifted and the reflexes coordinate the muscular activities required for complete emptying. The muscles, too, need to be strong enough for their jobs as a weak bladder will not be able to empty itself efficiently, and weak sphincters will not be able to prevent unwanted leakage of urine (see Figures 6a and 6b).

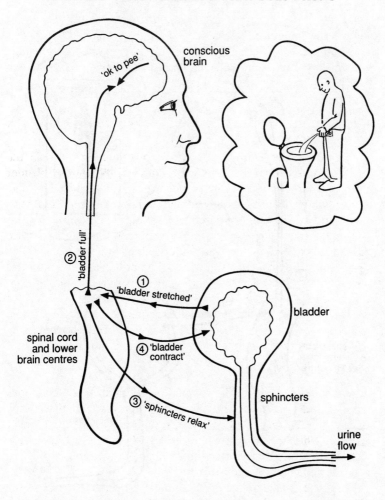

Fig. 6a A simplified model of the control system. The reflex centres in the spinal cord and lower brain can co-ordinate the action of the bladder muscle and sphincter muscles to empty the bladder efficiently without input from conscious levels of the brain.

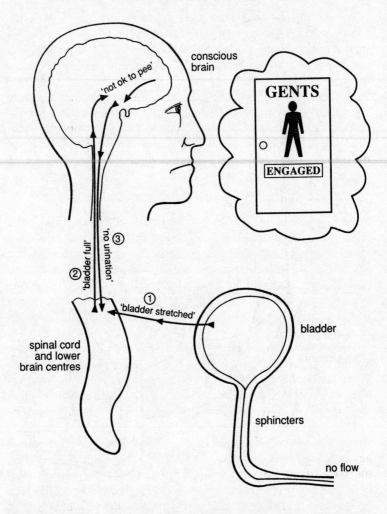

Fig. 6b When urination is not wanted, signals from the higher brain levels are transmitted to the lower centres to inhibit reflex emptying. The bladder remains relaxed and the sphincters remain contracted.

Problems in any facet of the system, from muscle injury to mental confusion, can cause difficulty, and emotional states are notorious for their effect on bladder control. 'I almost wet myself' applies to both very frightening and very funny events. A particularly common fault in the control system shows up as bladder instability. An unstable bladder contracts as if to expel urine at inappropriate times instead of remaining relaxed while it fills, and this produces a sensation of urgent need to pee. It can result from a habit of frequent emptying, from diseases affecting the controlling nerve pathways, from obstruction to the flow of urine or for no apparent reason at all.

What causes prostate enlargement?

So far, all we can say for certain is that being male and growing older are the key factors to prostate enlargement, and since you cannot avoid either you may feel that this information is less than useful! We *do* know which part of the prostate causes the trouble – the central part, close around the urethra – and we have a very strong suspicion that the male hormone testosterone is closely involved in the process, but we cannot say why some prostates enlarge so much earlier than others.

Studies have been done to compare the prevalence of prostate enlargement in different countries and in different groups of people in the same country, but they are extremely difficult to interpret because the number of cases diagnosed is not at all the same thing as the number of cases occurring. Some groups of men have very limited access to a doctor and other groups choose not to see one, while others tend to seek help very early. There are differences among doctors too, and they will not all give the same diagnosis for the, same symptoms. All these factors confuse the picture and, perhaps as a result, there is no convincing evidence to link the occurrence of benign prostate enlargement with racial background or with any aspect of lifestyle such as diet or smoking.

Since there is no clear evidence on which to base it, there is no advice to be given about how to avoid prostate enlargement, and no sense in reproaching yourself with thoughts of 'If only I had done x . . .' or 'I wouldn't be in this mess if I hadn't done y'. In fact, practically everyone would show the first microscopic signs of enlargement if they lived to be 100. The question the researchers are really trying to answer is, why do some men suffer at 50 while others survive unscathed to 90?

It seems quite clear that the answer has something to do with the male hormone testosterone. It is probably not a matter of the overall level of testosterone, which falls with advancing age equally in men with and without a prostate problem, but a question of what the prostate gland actually does with the testosterone reaching it. Enlarged prostates are suspected of converting testosterone into a particular derivative (5-alpha dihydrotestosterone) to a greater extent that normal prostates do, and it could be that this derivative promotes the enlargement. However, it also seems clear that the changes in the prostate which eventually lead to benign enlargement take place decades before the enlargement can be detected and no one knows yet what is going on at that initial stage.

The effect of prostate enlargement and outflow obstruction

Prostate enlargement is not a problem in itself. The problems only come when the prostate obstructs the flow of urine out of the bladder, and the degree of obstruction does not depend simply on the size of the prostate. Relatively small glands can cause severe obstruction if they are of just the wrong shape, while very large glands sometimes cause very little obstruction and need no treatment.

The symptoms are described here in the typical order in which they might occur but this does not mean that everyone will have all of them. It is possible for early symptoms to develop but never progress, and it is possible to have so-called late symptoms without ever having noticed any early warning signs.

Initial symptoms

The first symptoms – hesitancy and slow flow – are the direct result of obstruction. Obstruction may also cause intermittent flow and terminal dribble but this is less certain.

With the enlarged prostate pressing on the uretha, the bladder has to produce a higher pressure than normal to force it open and, because it takes a little time for the bladder to generate this pressure, there is a hesitation between getting ready to pee and the urine beginning to flow. If the pressure the bladder can produce is closely balanced with the obstructive pressure from the prostate, the urethra may shut during urination causing an intermittent flow. This is particularly likely towards the end of urination when the

22

pressure produced by the bladder falls away, and terminal dribble is a common early symptom. A slow flow of urine is very likely while the bladder keeps its old strength but struggles to empty through a constricted pipe.

At this stage, the bladder may still manage to empty itself completely. Sudden inability to pee at all can occur, but this is more likely to happen later after there has been an insidious build-up of retained urine.

The response of the bladder and subsequent symptoms

The later symptoms of urgency, frequency, nocturia and possibly incontinence come about as the bladder responds to the obstruction and as the obstruction progresses. These symptoms are variable as different bladders respond in different ways.

Hypertrophy and instability

Forcing out urine against an increased pressure means extra work for the bladder and, often, the bladder muscle responds like any other muscle to the increased workload by thickening and becoming stronger. This growth ('hypertrophy') enables the bladder to continue emptying itself despite the obstruction. At the same time, it often becomes unstable and contracts as if to empty itself before it is really full. The result is a frequent feeling of urgent need to pee, so that the dashes to the toilet become more and more numerous and more and more urgent. The frequency may extend to the night-time, causing nocturia, and the urgency may become so extreme that accidents happen on the way to the toilet.

The symptoms produced by these responses are distressing but there is some evidence that they are protective in that they delay the onset of urine retention and irreversible effects on the kidneys. The bladder muscle is retaining its strength and will be able to work effectively again if the obstruction is removed.

Decompensation and urine retention

Decompensation is a weakening of the bladder which happens when it becomes unable to empty properly. Some bladders seem to give up the struggle against obstruction very early, without ever strengthening in response. Others are eventually overwhelmed by the progressively increasing obstruction. Then the bladder no longer manages to empty itself completely. At first the amount of residual urine left behind is small but it increases gradually until there is a chronic retention of urine and the bladder is constantly stretched.

Usually, once urine is retained, frequency of urination and night-time peeing become a nuisance. The bladder can only hold a certain amount so if a large amount is always left after urination then obviously only a small amount can be released – and if you can only empty tiny amounts at a time, you will have to do so very frequently. Severe retention can also lead to incontinence. It is quite typical to lose a small amount of urine soon after falling asleep, and in the most extreme case overflow incontinence can occur where the bladder is always stretched to its maximum capacity and urine is forced out in a constant dribble.

The amount of urine retained can be enormous (up to ten pints or even more) so that the bladder muscle is stretched out very thinly and is severely weakened. It may not ever regain its strength fully, even after an operation to relieve the obstruction.

Against a background of chronic retention, quite minor additional factors can trigger a sudden complete retention of urine. Suspected causes include cold, alcohol and holding on too long, as well as certain drugs which are known to encourage the system to seize up even when it has previously been working well.

Effects on the kidneys and late symptoms

Problems for the kidneys begin if urine is retained at high pressure because, with urine at high pressure in the ureters, the normal pressure difference which allows the kidneys to filter the blood is diminished. Urine production is disrupted and the kidneys are unable to remove waste effectively from the blood or to regulate the levels of essential minerals correctly. Other functions of the kidney are also at risk, so anaemia and raised blood pressure may ensue, and kidney infection is another unwelcome possibility as bacteria can breed in the stagnant pool of urine.

Oddly, too much urine may be produced because the ability of the kidneys to produce concentrated urine is particularly sensitive to small degrees of damage. The urine may contain unusual ingredients such as proteins which would show that the filter itself is no longer working correctly.

If the disease progresses to this stage, the symptoms extend beyond the urinary system. Chief among them is a feeling of general malaise, lethargy and unwellness which may go along with headaches and feverish symptoms, pain in the kidney area and thirst. Treatment should begin as soon as possible.

The likely progression of the condition

An enlarged prostate is likely to carry on enlarging for several years, so the obstruction may worsen in that time and it is important to monitor the situation if it is not treated at once. However, the symptoms often vary from week to week and it is not inevitable that they will become very much worse over a period of, say, five years. There is a little more detail about this in Chapter 6, page 69.

Other conditions causing similar symptoms

Mostly, symptoms suggestive of enlarged prostate really are due to a benignly enlarged prostate. However, other possibilities range from the mundane (constipation) to the alarming (cancer), and from the common (bladder instability) to the unusual (stricture).

Cancer

Let's deal with cancer first, not because it is especially likely but because it is so feared. You should be aware that cancer is a possibility, and that this is one reason to take your symptoms to a doctor instead of putting up with them as an unavoidable aspect of your age, but you should keep the possibility in perspective. It is *possible* for an enlarged prostate to be malignant but it is much more *likely* to be benign.

Prostate cancer

Cancer as a whole becomes more common with increasing age and this is particularly true of prostate cancer, with half of the cases and well over half of the deaths occurring in men over the age of 75. Cancer of the prostate accounts for 10 per cent of all male cancers: one in twenty of those discovered in men between the ages of 45 and 64, one in ten of those found between 65 and 74, and one in six of those in men aged 75 or more. Translated into risks, this means that the chance of a man finding that he has prostate cancer in any one year is approximately 1 in 4000 between 45 and 64 years old, 1 in 500 between 65 and 74 and 1 in 200 at 75+. The disease is extremely rare under the age of 45.

Prostate cancer is less likely than benign enlargement at all ages but it will still be in your doctor's mind as a possibility because it can cause enlargement and obstruction, so the early symptoms can be practically indistinguishable.

Cancer and benign enlargement are quite separate entities and benign enlargement does not progress into cancer. Cancer generally develops in the outer part of the gland, while benign overgrowth arises in the central area. Having benign enlargement does not make it more likely that you will have prostate cancer, but it does make it more likely to be detected because pieces of the prostate removed during an operation will be examined very closely. Under such scrutiny, previously unsuspected cancer cells are found in about one case in eight. Other men of the same age are equally likely to have cancer cells in their prostates but those who do not have benign enlargement do not have operations and so do not find out about them. Some such cancers, only noticed incidentally at an operation, have little sinister potential and cause no harm. Autopsy studies show that many men (over half of those aged 80+) have had them without ever being aware of it.

Bladder cancer

Bladder cancer is less common than prostate cancer, accounting for about 7 per cent of cancers in men overall, and it is not likely to be confused with benign prostatic enlargement because it does not normally cause obstruction and the symptoms related to obstruction. The main warning signal is blood in the urine, which is why this symptom should always be taken seriously.

Bladder instability and related complaints

Bladder instability (see pages 21 and 23) is very common, affecting at least two in three men with outflow obstruction and about one in three men of similar age who have no obstruction. Bladder instability can be confused quite easily with prostate enlargement because it often leads to frequency and urgency of peeing, and sometimes incontinence and nocturia. It can even mimic slow stream because, if you empty very small amounts of urine, the flow does tend to be slow. Also, it often exists alongside prostate enlargement either as a result of obstruction or just as a co-incidence.

Most bladder instability is 'idiopathic' i.e. not a sign of anything else, simply existing of itself, but it becomes more common with increasing age, probably because the inevitable wear and tear on the nerves and brain weakens their control over the bladder muscle.

However, even when a stroke has injured the brain, it is often possible to retrain the bladder to hold a reasonable volume of urine and contract only when urination is required. Diseases which affect the workings of the nervous system such as longstanding diabetes, multiple sclerosis and Parkinson's disease make bladder instability more likely.

Dyssynergia is another form of nerve-muscle misbehaviour in which the bladder neck or sphincter fails to open when the bladder muscle contracts, and therefore the flow of urine is very slow. It is not particularly common and it takes very detailed testing to discover it.

Nocturnal polyuria

Nocturnal polyuria means production of a large volume of urine overnight and it inevitably means a number of night-time trips to the toilet. Apart from its effect on your sleep, it is harmless. Urine production may be normal or reduced by day so there are no daytime symptoms of frequency, urgency or slow stream and this allows a doctor to tell it apart from prostatic obstruction (so long as there is no other condition such as instability to confuse the picture).

Sometimes the overnight urine is removing fluid which had pooled in the lower legs during the day and came back into the main circulation when you lay down at night; this is likely if you do a lot of sitting during the day and little walking. Another possible cause is an alteration in the daily cycle of release of ADH, a hormone which normally ensures that urine production is reduced at night.

Urinary tract infection

Urinary tract infection usually means bacteria growing in the bladder or urethra, although the kidneys can be affected too and this is much more serious. Infection and inflammation often cause frequency and urgency of urination, and slow stream because of emptying small volumes at a time, but the symptom which stands out and differs from prostatic obstruction is a burning pain when peeing.

Urinary infection is unusual in men unless there is an obstruction to the flow of urine, or stones in the urinary tract, so it should be thoroughly investigated. Sometimes a sexually transmitted infection produces similar symptoms.

Prostatitis and related complaints

Inflammation of the prostate is not unusual and commonly occurs at an earlier age than prostate enlargement. Often a bacterial infection is the cause, and often the same bacteria cause urinary infections, but bacteria cannot always be detected when there are symptoms and sometimes bacteria are found when there are no symptoms.

The symptoms of prostatitis vary but include tenderness when the prostate is examined. There may be chills and fever, pain in the lower back and perineum (the 'saddle area'), and possibly frequency and pain in urination.

Not all pain in the perineal area is really due to prostatitis. Sometimes there is no cause that any doctor can find and it may be that, as with recurrent tension headaches, the cause actually lies elsewhere.

Stricture

A stricture is simply a narrowing of a passage, so the constriction produced by the enlarged prostate could be called a stricture, but in this book stricture only refers to other narrowings in the urethra. These usually follow from infection, with gonorrhoea for example, or from scarring due to accidental injury, or from the use of medical instruments passed through the urethra. Where the constriction is pronounced, the flow of urine is obstructed and this leads to the same sort of symptoms as prostate enlargement.

Stones

Stones, also called calculi, can form in the kidney, bladder or prostate (where they may be linked with prostatitis). Kidney stones are commoner than bladder stones: they would not be confused with prostate enlargement as their main symptom is severe pain in the loin. Bladder stones may show up by causing difficulty in passing urine, but very likely there would have been some difficulty in passing urine even before the stone formed as they seldom occur unless there is an obstruction to urine flow or a longstanding urinary infection.

Constipation

The upper part of the urethra and the prostate lie close to the front wall of the rectum. If you have constipation, the hard faeces in the rectum press on the wall making it bulge and constricting or

28

blocking the urethra. This produces an obstruction at very much the same level as an enlarged prostate would and, if it is longstanding, it can produce very similar symptoms. However, it should be detected simply enough on your first visit to a doctor and it can usually be treated without much difficulty.

Excessive drinking

If you drink a vast amount, you will have to pee a great deal, obviously, but it is quite easy to distinguish this frequency from the frequency due to an enlarged prostate because you should not have a poor stream of urine or any special urgency to reach the toilet. If you are drinking such a lot because you are really thirsty, there could be an illness at the root of it such as diabetes or poor kidney function which should be investigated. Otherwise, so long as the amount of alcohol in the drink is limited, it is not going to do any harm and it is not a sign of anything amiss.

Bad habit

If you get into a habit of emptying your bladder at the first hint of its filling, it is very easy to lose confidence in its ability to hold a normal amount. Soon, you find yourself using a toilet at every opportunity 'just in case' and what started as a habit becomes an escalating problem. Some workers believe that this can even lead to bladder instability. However, you can retrain your bladder (see page 112) and regain your confidence.

4

Medical Investigations

Why bother?

There is no need to worry just because you are getting up a couple of times a night for a pee. Apart from that, if your usual habits of bladder emptying have changed enough to notice, it is time to consult a doctor. Why?

First, you will probably guess that the cause of your symptoms is an enlarged prostate (a *benignly* enlarged prostate), and you will probably be right, and in the early stages it will probably do you little lasting harm. However, as you know from Chapter 3, there are other possible causes and the one which your doctor will be looking out for particularly is the possibility of prostate cancer which is amongst the commoner cancers in older men. Like all cancers, it is very much better to catch it early as it can be treated more effectively before it spreads. Incidentally, you may hear doctors referring to the enlargement of your prostate as an 'adenoma' (or perhaps a 'tumour'). This sounds scary because many cancers have names ending with -oma, but it does *not* mean that it is a malignant cancer. An adenoma means a tumour of a gland, and a tumour, strictly speaking, only means a swelling. A typical benign enlargement of the prostate is an adenoma.

A second reason to consult your doctor is that even benign enlargement can have serious consequences for your kidneys. Occasionally it progresses towards this stage before causing very notable symptoms. A doctor can use simple tests to tell if this is happening and arrange for prompt treatment.

Third, the symptoms themselves can be very distressing but in most cases, once the cause has been found, they can be treated. You do not have to expect to put up with them for the rest of your life.

Do not be put off by the fact that the doctor seems busy. Make an appointment, for a week or more ahead if necessary, rather than leave it and think you will come back when things are quieter. They never are quieter. Your needs are no less important than those of other patients, and you are certainly not wasting the doctor's time. Do not be put off by embarrassment either. No doctor will be embarrassed – they deal with this kind of thing every day – and they will be equally comfortable whether you talk of peeing, urinating, passing water or anything else. If you do feel diffident, you only need to decide how you are going to introduce the subject (e.g. 'I'm having trouble with my waterworks') and leave it to them to lead the discussion after that.

When you go to the doctor, he or she will ask you lots of questions, do various checks and probably send you on to the local hospital for more tests. The point of all these investigations, obviously, is to find out exactly what is wrong so that the best treatment can be chosen. There is no point, for instance, in having an operation to unblock the pipe unless a blockage in the pipe is really at the root of the trouble. Every investigation should add a piece of information which will make a difference in the decision about treatment. Some investigations are really essential for everyone, others are of little value except in certain circumstances. What is suggested will depend on the complexity of your case and the preferences of the professionals you come into contact with. They should be prepared to tell you, if you ask, what they are trying to find out and what difference that information could make – as well as exactly what is involved in the test from your point of view. You can refuse any investigation, of course, as your informed consent is needed for any medical procedure, not just for treatment.

Making the best of an appointment

Knowing what to expect during your appointment is a great help in making the best use of it. Then you can be prepared, both with answers for the doctor's questions and with any questions of your own.

You will know whether you are the sort of person who wants to be told everything about your condition so that you can make your own decisions, or whether you are the sort who prefers to delegate the decision-making to the professionals as far as possible and know only what it is essential to know. Your own doctor may know which sort you are, too, but the other doctors you meet will not and they may not volunteer information in case you are the delegating sort. However, most doctors are quite glad to give you answers when you ask sensible questions and show that you want to know.

It is a great help to write questions down beforehand as it is easy to get flustered, particularly in the unfamiliar environment of a hospital. If you read ahead in this book, more questions will occur to you. Is treatment necessary now, or would it be safe to wait a while? What options are there and what risks are attached? How big would you say those risks are in my particular case? Could I try bladder training in the meantime?

Providing that you feel at ease with him or her, it is usually best to go to your own family doctor who already knows you and understands your medical background. If you would prefer to see some other particular doctor, or a doctor of a particular sex, ask. You do not have a right to insist on it, but there is seldom any problem in seeing another member of the practice if your doctor works with a group. You can also express a preference about which specialist you are referred to, and you can refuse to be examined by, or in the presence of, students. Both men and women work in all areas of the Health Service these days, of course, so do not be surprised to find female doctors, surgeons and anaesthetists as well as male ones, and male nurses as well as female.

The rest of this chapter describes the main investigations which may be carried out, and the likeliest settings for them. However, there is some variation over who does which tests so, for example, blood tests and urine tests might equally well be done by your own doctor or in the hospital outpatient department. It is not likely that you will have all of the tests, but it is quite likely that you will have some – like the rectal examination – more than once, by different doctors, and it is almost certain that different doctors will ask you the same questions over again. This is irritating but at least they are not relying on increasingly garbled information passed on from one to another.

Investigations by your family doctor

General medical history

Your doctor will be interested in all your symptoms. How strong is the urine flow (how high up the wall can you pee?), do you have to wait for it to get started or for it to stop properly? Is there any pain when you urinate, any other pain, any discharge from your penis? How many times in the day do you empty your bladder, and how many times at night? Do you ever wet yourself? How are your symptoms affecting your life? How long have they been noticeable? It is worth working out the answer to this one before you go, as it can be hard to remember.

Be sure to mention any changes in your health which you have noticed, such as general tiredness or backache, even if they do not seem to you to be related to your bladder problem. Also, make sure that all the doctors know everything about your medical history which may be significant, even if it has not changed lately and even if they do not ask. For instance, anything which affects the health of your whole body is relevant, such as diabetes, haemophilia or penicillin allergy and any drugs you are taking regularly such as steroids for rheumatoid arthritis, antidepressants or heart pills. Anything which affects your heart is relevant to surgery, such as having a pacemaker or having had rheumatic heart disease. Anything to do with your pelvic area is relevant, such as once having had a fractured pelvis or a pelvic operation, or having a hydrocoele or a tight foreskin. Future medical plans are relevant, too, such as being scheduled for a hip replacement operation. All of these things may influence the decision about whether to operate, how to operate and when to operate.

Rectal examination

The doctor can feel the prostate where it presses against the front wall of the rectum. Part of the point of doing so is to check its size, although finding that it is enlarged does not prove that this is the cause of the trouble. Most older men have enlarged prostates and many of them have no symptoms. On the other hand, you can have quite a severe obstruction with a relatively small prostate. Another part of the point of the rectal examination is to check that the prostate has a normal texture despite its size and is not obviously cancerous. Finally, it may be that chronic constipation is causing or contributing to the problem; a rectal examination will find this and your own doctor will be able to offer treatment for it (see Figure 7).

The doctor needs to insert a finger into your back passage. Men I have spoken with comment that this is distasteful or disagreeable or undignified, rather than actually painful. It is best for you if you can relax so that the muscles around your anus do not tense up and make it more uncomfortable than it need be. The doctor, of course, has done this examination dozens of times before and is not embarrassed on his own account. He wears very light plastic gloves and uses a slippery gel on his finger for lubrication. You lie on your side with your legs curled up slightly.

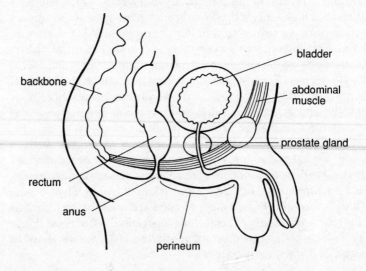

Fig. 7 A side view from the right showing how close the prostate is to the front wall of the rectum. You can also see how an overfilled bladder would press against the muscles of the abdominal wall.

Abdominal examination

If you have a lot of urine remaining in your bladder after peeing, that is a large residual volume or chronic retention, the doctor can discover this by feeling your abdomen.

Blood pressure

Not all doctors feel that it is necessary to measure blood pressure when investigating straightforward urinary symptoms. If the disease had gone so far as to cause kidney damage, that in turn could cause raised blood pressure, but the kidney damage would be detected by a urine or blood test in any case. However, raised blood pressure is always worth detecting, and the test is extremely simple, so it is quite sensible for doctors to measure it whenever they get the chance.

Urine tests

You can learn a lot from urine. You could take a sample (a *small* fresh sample!) with you in a clean bottle, or your doctor may give you a specimen bottle to fill at your leisure and hand in later for testing. You should take your sample when your flow is well started, not right at the beginning or end, and hand it in for testing within an hour of producing it.

Simple tests with chemical dipsticks in the doctor's surgery can show if the urine contains sugar, which might indicate diabetes, or protein, which might indicate bladder infection or poor working in the kidneys. The hospital laboratory can culture the urine on jelly to see whether it contains bacteria and, if so, which antibiotics they are sensitive to; this takes a few days. Urine always contains some cells from the bladder wall and these can be examined under a microscope to see whether they look normal. At the same time, the microscopist would notice any red cells which would show that blood was present in the urine.

Whether it is done by your family doctor or later at the hospital clinic, a urine test must be done at some stage.

A related test is called EPS, meaning expressed prostatic secretion. This involves taking urine samples before and after massaging the prostate (by way of the rectum), and it aims to find bacteria sheltering in the prostate. It is not done routinely.

Investigations by clinic or specialist

Unless your symptoms are mild and your doctor is sure that there is nothing seriously amiss, he will usually refer you to a specialist in a hospital. Ask what sort of specialist this is. Urologists (specialists in urinary matters), on the whole, feel that prostate surgery is best done by specialist urological surgeons and not by general surgeons, as the hollowing out of the prostate with fine telescopic instruments inserted through the penis must be done very accurately and it is a technique unlike other surgical techniques. Also, a urologist is more likely to be familiar with non-surgical treatments which can be more appropriate than an operation in some cases. However, in some areas it may be customary to refer patients to general surgeons or to general surgeons with a particular interest in urological matters. You can query this.

Your next stop may be a clinic which carries out various tests before sending you to the specialist with the results, or a specialist who talks to you and examines you before sending you off for further tests. Whatever the organization of the system, you should not be listed for surgery until you have had tests which show definite evidence of obstruction. At least 70 per cent of men over 60 have some urinary symptoms or some prostate enlargement, or both, but they do not all have obstruction and they do not all need surgery. One study published in 1990 showed that one in four men who had been placed on a waiting list for prostatectomy purely on the basis of their symptoms in fact had no obstruction. In the absence of objective testing they would have gone on to have totally pointless operations.

Flow tests

These are very simple. You pee into a toilet fitted with electronic gadgetry which measures the volume of urine and the flow rate. The highest flow rate is the significant measurement. If it is below a certain level, it is highly likely that the outflow from your bladder is obstructed, so likely that it is hardly necessary to do any more tests for obstruction. Above a certain level, obstruction is not very likely to be the cause of the problem and the doctors will look for some other explanation. Between the two is a grey area where it may be worth doing more detailed 'urodynamic' tests.

It is important to do the test with your bladder as full as you can manage as the results are unreliable for very small urine volumes. The maximum flow rates depend on the total volume of urine produced as well as on your age, the strength of your bladder muscle and the severity of any obstruction there may be.

Flow tests are not perfectly foolproof because a low flow may be due to weakness of the bladder muscle, not obstruction, and a very strong bladder muscle can produce a reasonable flow rate despite an obstructed urethra, but they work very well in practice. The 1990 study mentioned above indicates that their use alone would cut the proportion of pointless prostatectomies ten-fold.

Bladder charts

Bladder charts, or frequency-volume charts, are even simpler than flow tests and give equally valuable information, although they will not prove the presence or absence of obstruction. The only special equipment needed is a measuring jug, as sold in hardware or kitchen shops, so you do not even need to wait for a doctor to arrange this test for you.

What you do is this: for one week, each time you pee, use the jug to measure the volume of urine you produce (preferably in millilitres (ml), but fluid ounces will do). Make a note of the time and volume each time. If you have any mishaps with your bladder control make a note of these too, with a W (for wet) or some other code; include something to jog your memory about the circumstances of the accident, such as being asleep or stuck in a traffic jam. You can draw this up as a chart, or simply write it as a list on a sheet of paper. Include a note of your bedtime and getting-up time.

There is a lot you or your doctor can learn from a chart like this. A 'normal' chart would show something like four to six toilet visits during the day, perhaps one at night, and a volume varying between about 200 and 400 ml each time. Of course, there is a lot of variation between healthy people, and from day to day, and the chart will reflect what you drink as well as the state of your kidneys and bladder, but there are several recognizable alterations from the normal pattern.

For example, if you add up the total volume of urine you produce during the night-time and compare it with the amount you produce during the daytime, you may find that your kidneys are, rather perversely, producing more urine at night. If you are producing, say, two pints (1200 ml) of urine overnight then it is really not the fault of your bladder or prostate that you have to get up three or four times to deposit it in the toilet; anyone would. Another fairly typical pattern is to go to the toilet very frequently during the day and produce small volumes of urine, but to sleep all night and produce a normal half pint or so (300–400 ml) in the morning. This goes to show that your bladder is physically capable of holding and emptying normal volumes but that something is interfering with this process while you are awake. Bladder instability can cause this pattern, and bladder training may be an appropriate treatment for it (see Chapter 8, page 112).

If your frequent bladder emptying is really caused by an enlarged prostate blocking the flow, you would expect to find frequent emptying of small volumes both day and night, although the frequency would be less severe during the night providing that your kidneys were behaving in the usual way and producing less urine than during the day.

Blood tests

It is routine to measure the amount of haemoglobin in blood. Haemoglobin is essential for carrying oxygen around your body, and a low haemoglobin level is one form of anaemia; it leaves you feeling weak and tired the whole time. There are all sorts of reasons for the haemoglobin level to be below normal, ranging from kidney damage to insufficient iron in your diet, but the cause should always be sought and treated.

Another test which is routine before surgery is blood grouping. It does not matter that you already know what blood group you are. The doctors will always insist on checking it although, in fact, there is a lot more to blood than its group and, if you do ever need to be given blood, the laboratory staff will not simply choose blood of the same group as yours. Except in the direst emergency, they will test your blood directly with the blood they are thinking of giving you to make sure that they do not react badly together.

The next test is to measure the amounts of waste chemicals in your blood such as urea and creatinine. These should be removed by the kidneys so high levels indicate that your kidneys are not working as well as they should be.

Finally, in many hospitals, blood will be tested for PSA (prostate specific antigen) or other substances which are made chiefly or exclusively by cells in the prostate. If there are high levels of these it may suggest that some prostate cells are overactive, possibly cancerous.

All sorts of other tests can be done on blood such as counting the different types of cells, looking at them microscopically, and measuring the levels of various substances relating to the activity of different organs. A doctor will not ask for all of these to be done, only those which are likely to be relevant to your illness. If you are interested in what may be done, or what has been done and what the results mean, *ask*.

X-rays

It is quite common to have a simple x-ray of your abdomen with the x-ray beam angled to show up your kidneys, ureters and bladder. This is often called a 'KUB' in jargon. It will detect any major abnormalities such as stones in your bladder or kidneys, and although the shadows of the kidneys and bladder are rather hazy to an inexperienced eye, a specialist can get a good idea of whether a large volume of urine is remaining in the bladder after you have tried to empty it.

The x-ray dose is very small for a plain film like this.

Intravenous urography or pyelography

Intravenous pyelography (IVP) is the same thing as intravenous urography (IVU). It is an x-ray investigation which involves injecting a contrast-medium – a chemical which shows clearly on x-ray photographs – into your blood. The contrast-medium is excreted by the kidneys and x-rays are taken at intervals over the next one to four hours until it has passed through the system completely. This technique produces clear pictures of the kidneys, ureters and bladder but it has disadvantages and it is widely agreed that it should not be used routinely.

Several x-rays are taken so the x-ray dose is higher than with a single plain picture. More importantly, there are risks attached to the use of the contrast-medium – one in two thousand of having a reaction to it which needs medical treatment, one in forty thousand of dying as a result. Those are very small risks, but it is not worth taking them unless the procedure is going to produce useful information. In practice, in straightforward cases, the chance of finding out anything which will influence the choice of treatment is very small.

There is some reason to have intravenous urography if you have had blood in your urine, or a history of kidney disease or severe infection in the urinary system. Otherwise, query the need for it.

Ultrasound and the measurement of residual urine

A large volume of urine remaining in your bladder is clearly abnormal and it is usually considered a good reason to operate without excessive delay. It is logical to suppose that the stagnant urine will provide a breeding ground for bacteria and make you prone to urinary infections, and there is a concern that an overfilled bladder may allow urine to back up the inflow pipes and affect the workings of the kidneys.

There are several ways to measure residual urine. One is by intravenous urography, discussed above. Another is by passing a fine tube into the bladder through the penis and measuring the volume of urine which flows out; this might be done along with urodynamic studies (discussed shortly). Some doctors feel that the bladder shadow on a plain x-ray gives them a good enough idea of the amount of urine remaining, and say that routine ultrasound – the chosen method in many clinics – is just as un-necessary as routine urography, though safer.

An ultrasound examination is straightforward from the patient's point of view, involving nothing more than a small device pressed onto the skin of your abdomen with a little soft jelly to improve the acoustic contact. The picture shows up on a TV screen at the time, and the operator measures the diameter of the bladder in order to calculate the volume. She can also obtain a picture of your kidneys by placing the head of the machine between the lower ribs on your back.

Urodynamic tests

Urodynamic tests, also called video pressure-flow studies or videocystourethrography, give the most detailed understanding of the workings of your bladder, urethra and sphincters (tank, pipe and taps). Cystometry is similar, measuring the pressure in the bladder as it is filled, but less extensive.

A very slender catheter is passed through the urethra, and a tiny pressure transducer is passed through this into the bladder. Another pressure transducer is placed in the rectum. Measuring the pressure in both places allows the effect of bladder muscle activity, which only affects the bladder pressure, to be seen separately from the effect of other activities such as coughing or changing position which alter the pressure in the rectum as well as in the bladder.

The pressures are measured while the bladder is filled with liquid via the catheter. The filling liquid can be a contrast-medium; it will not have the same dangers as in intravenous urography as it does not go into the bloodstream. Then the catheter can be removed and the pressures measured while you empty your bladder; the rate of flow can also be measured as in simple flow studies. Finally, the pressure at different points along the urethra can be measured as the pressure transducer is pulled out, showing how effectively the sphincters can shut off the urethra and prevent urine flow. During each of these phases, video recordings of the bladder and urethra can be made.

At the end of all this, the doctors will know whether your bladder stays at low pressure as it should while it fills, or whether the pressure rises unduly. They will know whether it has waves of unintended and irrepressible activity, i.e. whether it is unstable. They will know whether it can produce sufficient pressure to empty itself, or whether it has been so stretched that it has lost its strength, and they will know how much urine remains in the bladder after emptying. If there is an obstruction in the outflow, they will know where it is. They will be able to see if urine makes its way in the wrong direction up the tubes to the kidneys, or into abnormal pouches (diverticula) in the bladder wall. In fact, there is very little that is left unknown.

Full-scale urodynamic testing is the Rolls Royce of urological investigations and, like a Rolls Royce, best kept for special occasions. It is time-consuming and expensive, not particularly enjoyable for most patients, and it often gives more detail than is really needed. In a straightforward case where the symptoms are typical of prostatic obstruction, where a rectal examination shows an enlarged prostate, and simple flow tests show that there is an obstruction, it is not necessary to have full urodynamic tests.

Like other examinations, urodynamic studies are more undignified than uncomfortable, but they are everyday work so far as the staff are concerned. The best attitude for the patient is probably one of curiosity rather than embarrassment; you seldom get a chance to see the workings of your body in such fascinating detail. Afterwards, you may find that you feel a need to empty your bladder even more often than usual. This is because the catheter irritates the smooth lining of the urethra. Drink plenty of water to keep the urine dilute and the feeling should pass off within a day or two. If not, see your own doctor to make sure that you have not picked up an infection.

Transrectal ultrasound

Transrectal ultrasound is not a routine investigation but its use is becoming more widespread. By placing an ultrasound transducer in the rectum, where it is very close to the prostate, an accurate picture of the prostate can be obtained. Most prostates can safely be removed via the penis without making any incision but very large ones are better taken out through a cut in the abdomen, so the picture is useful for measuring the size of the prostate in order to plan the best route for surgery. A more important use is to detect small nodules of cancer inside the gland which cannot be felt with a finger.

Prostatic needle biopsy

Biopsies are only done if there is a reason to suspect cancer. A sample of prostate tissue is taken with a needle inserted from the rectum, and examined microscopically to see if the cells appear malignant. An ultrasound picture may be used at the same time, to guide the sampling needle to the areas that look most suspicious.

Biopsies are unpleasant, but they should only be done when they are really necessary – i.e. when cancer is suspected but not yet proved, and would be treated if found. Treatment for cancer is no holiday itself, and no one would undertake it without being certain that cancer was really present.

Investigations before operation

ECG chest x-ray

ECG (Electrocardiography, a trace and print-out of the heart's activity) and chest x-ray are straightforward checks which are usually done in hospital very shortly before surgery, although the x-ray might be done in an outpatients' department a week or two earlier. They are described briefly in Chapter 7 (page 91).

Cystoscopy

Cystoscopy means looking at the inside of the urethra and bladder through a tube with a light source and a lens system. It is usually the very last check to be done, when you are finally anaesthetized and ready for surgery. It would only be done earlier if there was some reason to think that there was another disease present which had not been clearly identified by any of the other tests.

Histology

Histology means microscopic examination of samples of tissue. After prostatectomy, samples of the tissue cut out from the prostate will always be examined in this way to look for signs of cancer. It is not unusual to find a few abnormal cells – it depends largely on just how hard you look – but it does not mean that you should panic. There are different degrees of malignancy, and your consultant will talk to you about what treatment would be most appropriate. If the abnormal cells are few and not very malignant-looking, it may be best to leave well alone. They are not likely to cause real trouble in the time available, and the operation may already have removed them all anyway.

5
Choice of Treatment

This chapter describes the treatment which you are likely to be offered – in enough detail to let you make a reasonably informed choice between them. It also gives a brief outline of treatments which are as yet experimental, or at least unconventional, such as treatment by lasers or microwaves.

If you are offered a non-standard treatment, find out about it before you accept. What advantage is it supposed to have over the usual treatments? What is known of its side-effects? What is known of its long-term effectiveness? Will it interfere with the success of other treatments if these become necessary? The most usual treatment, prostatectomy, is not perfect but at least it has been in use for long enough to be fairly well understood.

When you are thinking about what treatments to take, make sure that your information is up-to-date and accurate. Do not rely on anecdotes and old memories. You may remember your grandfather having an operation and having a very hard time of it – but that was fifty years ago, and things have changed. Your friends may tell you more recent horror stories – but do not assume that these give the typical picture: the one story where things go wrong is always more interesting to tell than the nine where recovery is complete and uneventful. If you have particular worries, discuss them with your doctor or specialist, even if they seem a bit silly; he should have the sense to recognize that the worry is real whether or not it is well-founded, and he should take the trouble to explain the situation to you accurately.

It is, of course, essential to know exactly what is wrong before deciding how to treat it, which is why the investigations described in Chapter 4 are so important.

Treatment of benign prostate enlargement

There are four likely options for the treatment of a benignly enlarged prostate: no treatment (which doctors are more likely to call conservative treatment or watchful waiting), surgical treatment, drug treatment and treatment with a mechanical device, i.e. a catheter or stent.

The choice of which is most appropriate depends on how severe the problem is in medical terms (whether it is threatening vital systems such as your kidneys, for instance), your general state of health and any other illnesses you may have. It also depends very much on your personal assessment of the problem, and of the risks and benefits of the treatment. You are the only one who knows how much the symptoms bother you, and so you are the only one who can decide what risks you are prepared to take in order to be rid of them. Would it be worth a one in a hundred risk of incontinence, for example?

Watchful waiting

The great advantage of watchful waiting is that it is very unlikely to cause harm, it has no unexpected side-effects, and you can go on to another treatment at any time. If you can put up with your symptoms for a while longer, and there is no immediate medical reason for more active treatment, watchful waiting may be a good choice as there are disadvantages in going on to surgery too soon.

You are not necessarily going to get worse while you wait as, although the prostate will probably continue to grow for some time, the degree of obstruction may not change a great deal. The symptoms fluctuate so you will probably feel better at some times and worse at others. Studies looking at men treated (or untreated) in this way show that five years later less than half (10–40 per cent) have needed surgery and about half feel that their symptoms are the same or better. Bladder training (see Chapter 8, page 112) and drug treatment (see page 54) may help you to diminish the symptoms; these are possibilities to discuss with a doctor.

Being watchful, on your part, means being aware of your symptoms and being prepared to go back to your doctor if they worsen noticeably. Ideally, it should also mean having regular simple checks, especially of your flow rate. You could ask your specialist whether he thinks that this would be advisable or possible in the local situation.

Watchful waiting is clearly not a suitable strategy if the disease is already affecting your general health, or if it is likely to do so soon, so a doctor would probably recommend more vigorous treatment if you have blood in your urine, chronic retention or signs of kidney disorder. Active treatment is also probably advisable if you have very marked hesitancy, as this is a pointer to the likelihood of acute retention, and certainly if the prostate enlargement has already caused one episode of acute retention, as it is likely to do so again.

Surgical treatment

Surgery is the most favoured of the active treatments, 'the treatment of choice', and within surgical treatments the most favoured operation is called transurethral resection of the prostate, often abbreviated to TURP. This is a prostate removal (prostatectomy) done by way of the urethra, without making any incisions through the skin. In a few cases an open prostatectomy may be preferred, the prostate being removed through a cut. There are several slight variants of open prostatectomy depending on the exact site of the incision and the route taken from there to the prostate. These include retropubic (the most common), suprapubic, transvesical and perineal (extremely rare these days).

Prostatectomy

In 90 per cent of men, prostatectomy is done by way of the penis (transurethral resection). An open operation is needed for the other 10 per cent either because the prostate is unusually large, or because there are other problems, such as bladder stones to be dealt with at the same time, or very occasionally because of a difficulty like severe arthritis making it impossible for the patient to get into the position required for the transurethral operation. The results of the two operations are broadly similar, but open prostatectomy is a more major operation so you would feel worse for longer than after the typical transurethral prostatectomy.

The rest of this section focuses on the typical operation.

OUTLINE OF TYPICAL PROSTATECTOMY The surgeon uses a narrow tubular instrument fitted with viewing, cutting and sealing equipment which can be inserted through the natural opening of the penis. When it reaches the level of the prostate, the gland is cut away in small pieces from the inside (like coring an apple) and the pieces are washed away by a continuous flow of sterile fluid. Afterwards, a plastic tube (catheter) is left in place for a few days (see Figures 8a and 8b).

The operation is classed as a major one and it takes 6–12 weeks afterwards before you feel entirely yourself again. However, it is not particularly painful and the hospital stay itself is usually just

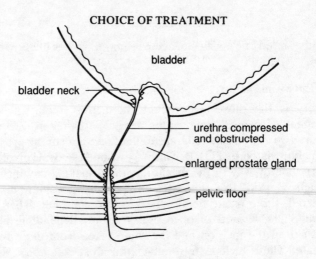

a { shows the areas with effective sphincter muscle

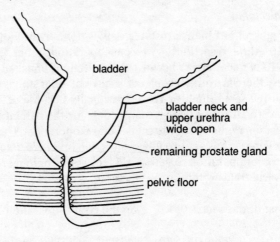

b { shows the areas with effective sphincter muscle

Fig. 8 Schematic side view of the bladder, prostate and upper urethra before and after prostatectomy showing the effect of the operation on the constriction and on the sphincter muscle. **a** Before: the enlarged prostate constricts the urethra and bulges into the bladder. **b** After: the bladder neck and upper urethra are left permanently open by the removal of the bulk of the prostate gland. The lower sphincter area is left intact or almost so.

under a week. For more detail about the practicalities of the operation and the recovery from it, see Chapters 7 and 8.

SUCCESS The chances are good that the operation will be a success. The success rate is 80 per cent looked at by men with an eye to the relief of their symptoms, and over 90 per cent looked at by doctors with an eye to the relief of obstruction. In other words, if the prostate gland is causing an obstruction, prostatectomy is almost certain to clear it, and four out of five men having a prostatectomy are pleased with the result.

There are various causes of dissatisfaction for the one in five men who are less than happy with the results. Some should not have had an operation in the first place, because the prostate was not actually the cause of the trouble; hence the importance of thorough investigations before surgery. A few have had technical failures where, although the prostate was the cause of obstruction, the operation failed to clear it; a repeat operation may solve the problem for them. Others continue to have symptoms although the underlying obstruction has been dealt with, and others again are unhappy with some side-effects of the operation. The question of success in curing particular symptoms is covered in the next paragraph, and side-effects in the following section.

The obstructive symptoms are very likely to be relieved by prostatectomy, with hesitancy, intermittent flow and poor stream cured in 85–90 per cent of cases. Frequency and peeing more than twice at night, with a cure rate of 70 per cent, are a little more recalcitrant, although the one in three chance that they will remain after prostatectomy is unsurprising in a way since about one in three of *all* men aged 60 to 85 have these symptoms. Urge incontinence (not a very common symptom anyway) shows a similar cure rate of about 70 per cent. The most persistent symptoms are urgency and after-dribble; the odds of curing these are about evens. Haemorrhoids (piles) which you probably think of quite separately from your prostate trouble are also likely to ease after prostatectomy.

SIDE-EFFECTS, SEX AND FERTILITY If you have enjoyed an active sex life before your operation, you can expect this to continue afterwards, although it will not be exactly the same as before. Some couples find the change an improvement, others are disappointed; it is a matter of preference.

The one predictable side-effect of prostatectomy, which occurs in about 80 per cent of men, is that, although you still have a satisfying orgasm, the sperm is no longer ejaculated out through your penis. The testicles continue to work perfectly well and produce sperm in the usual way but instead of the semen going forwards down your urethra to the outside, it goes backwards up the urethra into your bladder.

The backfiring of semen ('retrograde ejaculation' in medical jargon) happens because it is usually impossible to remove the obstructing part of the prostate without also removing the muscle which normally contracts and blocks off the bladder neck during intercourse. It does no harm to you, your penis or your bladder, but it does alter the sensation of orgasm and it does mean that your partner is unlikely to become pregnant. Even if you continue to ejaculate in the usual way after your operation, you are still likely (but not certain) to be infertile as sperms are absent from the fluid more often than not.

If you want to have more children – or think that you may want to in the future – the best option is to 'bank' sperm before the operation. This involves producing sperm (by masturbation) which is then deep frozen and stored. It is not guaranteed to be successful – not all sperm take kindly to being frozen – but it does give you a good chance.

Sperm banking services are very rarely available on the NHS, and only patchily available in the private sector, and the situation is changing rapidly as a result of legislation which requires centres offering assisted conception services to register with a central authority. You need to find out what is available now in your own area, or in an area you are prepared to travel to. It is simply a matter of telephoning hospitals and asking, but it may be a long chase so be prepared to be persistent. You can start with local hospitals, particularly any known for their maternity or fertility work, or with the national offices of the major private healthcare companies (AMI, Nuffield, BUPA etc.), or with a list of the centres registered with the Human Fertilization and Embryology Authority. An NHS hospital offering a private service in early 1992 was charging £50 for the initial freezing of the semen and £10 per year for the subsequent storage.

On the other hand, if you want a permanent form of contraception so that you can enjoy sex without any worry about a possible pregnancy, you cannot rely on prostatectomy to achieve this. An estimated 5–10 per cent of men retain some fertility afterwards.

Discuss the question of vasectomy (male sterilization) with your surgeon. This is a minor operation which can very easily be done at the same time as prostatectomy. You must continue to use a suitable contraceptive afterwards until your semen has been checked and confirmed to be sperm-free.

COMPLICATIONS Around four men in five have a straightforward recovery from the operation with no complications at all. A very small number have serious complications of the sort that could result from any operation – embolism in the lung or infection spreading to the blood for example. Amongst the rest, complications range from the relatively minor and temporary, such as urinary infections, to more serious problems such as strictures which require further surgery to set them right.

Mortality The most serious possible complication is death. It is uncommon as a result of prostatectomy, but all surgery carries risks and this operation is no exception. Many studies report death rates but the figures vary a great deal depending on which patients were selected for operation, how long they were followed up for, and whether the death rate is reported 'crude' or corrected for the men who would have died anyway even without an operation. The average death rate for all men having prostatectomy is not a very useful figure in any case. It does not tell you how safe the operation is for any one individual; it really tells you what risks people are prepared to take. As surgery becomes safer, men who would previously have been considered too frail for operation are accepted for surgical treatment. The result is that more, and sicker, men are treated and the overall death rates remain very much the same.

What you want to know is the risk for you individually, and your own surgeon and anaesthetist are best placed to advise you. They should be aware of all the relevant factors in your health, and they should know their own record with similar patients. As a guide, if you are relatively young (under 75), in good health and having your operation before the need for it becomes urgent, the chance of your dying as a result of it is very small indeed, less than one in five hundred. On the other hand, if you are older (over 85), have other health problems such as a previous heart attack (especially within the last six months), and if your prostate problem has progressed to the extent of causing acute or chronic retention, the risk of dying is considerable, perhaps as high as one in ten.

Impotence Impotence is *not* a common result of prostatectomy, and where it does happen it sometimes seems to be for psychological reasons. For example, if you believe that you are likely to be impotent, you may be afraid to try intercourse, or your anxiety itself may interfere with your erections – a classic self-fulfilling prophecy. Perhaps this is why one doctor has found that patients who are given no information about the sexual aspects of prostatectomy often believe that they are impotent afterwards, while those given a reassuring explanation beforehand continue to have happy sex.

Accidents are possible in surgery, of course, but the chance of causing physical impotence in a modern operation for benign enlargement of the prostate is small. The story is different with radical prostatectomy for cancer, a much more extensive operation which often did cause impotence, although a recent modification has improved the outlook. You should be sceptical over any horror stories you hear; they most probably relate to outdated versions of the operation, or to a different operation altogether.

Incontinence Incontinence is not uncommon in the first weeks after surgery, and at that time it is not so much a complication as an unpleasant aspect of recovery. Figures for permanent incontinence following prostatectomy vary from one study to another depending on how wide a definition the workers use. The risk of minor incontinence resulting from the operation is probably less than one in twenty, and the risk of severe incontinence around one in a hundred. Minor incontinence would mean occasional loss of urine, perhaps with physical activity or with a particularly urgent need to pee, while major incontinence would mean regular or continuous loss.

When incontinence does occur, it is usually because of a combination of an unstable bladder and weakness in the sphincter mechanism. Sphincter weakness can be due to injury, perhaps in an accident or previous surgery, or to deterioration in the nerves controlling the sphincter muscles, as might happen in longstanding diabetes, multiple sclerosis or a stroke. If you have one of these risk factors (previous pelvic fracture, surgery, diabetes, etcetera), there is a greater chance of your suffering incontinence after the operation. Make sure that your specialist is aware of it and discuss the risks carefully before deciding whether to go ahead with surgery or to try some other approach.

50

Stricture Strictures are narrowings in the urethra and they can occur when the urethra has been injured and scarred. About one in twenty men forms a stricture after prostatectomy, presumably because the instruments passed through the urethra have caused some damage. They usually take several months to develop, maybe more. Most strictures can be cured quite readily by another, much simpler, operation.

Bleeding Prostatectomy leaves a raw area where the prostate used to be which cannot be stitched up. A certain amount of bleeding is inevitable and no cause for alarm, but the medical staff will be watching carefully for excessive bleeding. This can happen immediately after the operation, or later when scabs break away. There is a chance of about one in twenty of bleeding severely enough to need treatment, which may include blood transfusion.

Urinary infections Urinary infections are common in the first three months after the operation, while the cut surface heals, especially if the bladder was already harbouring bacteria before the operation. The infections are not normally too troublesome but it is important to treat them with antibiotics to make sure that they do not spread while your defences are weakened by the stress of surgery. It is also helpful to keep up a good intake of watery drinks to keep flushing the bacteria out of the bladder.

Catheter problems Problems with the catheter used after surgery (see page 98) are seldom serious. About one in twenty men are unable to pee normally when the catheter is first removed a few days later. The catheter is then replaced for a day or so and most men are able to pee freely at the second attempt. A very small proportion have to be sent home with the catheter in place to have another try later still. Sometimes clots of blood or pieces of debris jam in the urethra after the catheter is removed, blocking the flow of urine again. This is unpleasant, but usually easily solved by the re-insertion of a catheter for a short time.

Transurethral resection syndrome The transurethral resection syndrome may happen if a large amount of the fluid used to wash away the fragments of prostate is absorbed into the bloodstream. The sudden influx overwhelms the body's mechanisms for keeping a proper chemical balance and produces nasty symptoms such as nausea, confusion and chest pains. This can be a very serious complication but it is rare, occurring in 1–2 per cent of operations.

Collapse of morale No research paper deals with collapse of morale as a complication, but it is well recognized by surgeons and nurses as one of the three commonest problems in the first few days after operation, along with bleeding and infection, and the hardest of the three to treat. Your best defence is to be well-informed about what to expect (see Chapters 7 and 8). Your bladder control will not be perfect immediately after the operation: you will have frequency and urgency and probably a number of accidents when you cannot reach the toilet quickly enough. This is a normal temporary phase. It will pass. Tissues heal, infections subside, the bladder gets over the disturbance of surgery. Control and confidence will return.

REPEAT OPERATIONS There is more chance (3–5 per cent) of needing a repeat operation in the first year after surgery than in any other year, presumably because some operations are incomplete and need to be finished off properly. However, even when the operation is as complete as it can be, an amount of the prostate gland is left behind and there is a possibility for the remainder to grow again and cause another obstruction in later years.

The estimates for how likely this is vary but the chance of needing another operation within five years is somewhere between one in ten and one in fifteen, and it does not seem to change as time goes on so there is the same chance again in the following five years. This means that in ten years, the possibility of needing another operation is somewhere between one in five and one in seven. The chance is significant but not overwhelming. Even extrapolating over 25 years, it is more likely than not that your first operation will be your only one.

DECIDING ON SURGERY The timing of an operation is important. If you have it too early, while the symptoms are relatively slight, the chance of relieving the symptoms is smaller and the chance of needing a repeat operation is higher. On the other hand, if you leave it too late the prostate problem may have affected your health so much that the operation itself is risky, or your bladder may have been so stretched for so long that it is unable to recover its strength even when the obstruction is removed.

Age in itself is no bar to having surgery and, occasionally, men of over 100 have had successful prostatectomies. More important than age is your general health, and the length of life ahead of you. Will your life be improved by enough and for long enough to make the risks and temporary discomforts of surgery worthwhile?

The decision to have, or not to have, surgery is yours in the end. There is a certainty of some temporary nuisance with it, a small chance of unwelcome side-effects, a good chance of relieving your symptoms. The doctors can tell you all this, they can perhaps put figures on the chances, but they cannot finally tell you whether it is worth it *to you*.

Other forms of surgery

The only operations in regular use for benign prostatic enlargement are the two sorts of prostatectomy – transurethral resection of the prostate and open prostatectomy. If you are offered any other sort of operation, treat it as experimental unless your specialist can convince you otherwise. I do not mean to put you off possible new treatments by saying this, as they could be very beneficial. I am just suggesting that if a treatment is not well established, you should be aware of that fact and its implications. Ask how thoroughly the method has been tested, and what is known of its possible risks and benefits.

If the proposed treatment is less major than a prostatectomy and expected to have smaller risks and fewer side-effects, you may be happy to try it, especially if you are not well enough for a traditional prostatectomy, or if you are particularly anxious to avoid its side-effects. If the operation is thought to be similar in scale to prostatectomy, it is sensible to be more cautious. What are its expected advantages, to outweigh the disadvantages of its being less well understood?

MICROWAVE HYPERTHERMIA The use of hyperthermia – raised temperature – to damage the prostate and cause it to shrink is not a new idea but it has been applied more effectively since the development of small microwave sources. At first, the microwave source was placed in the rectum but now that even smaller instruments have been designed it can be placed in the urethra and this gives better results. The aim is to produce a temperature of 45°C, compared with the normal body temperature of 37°C.

The treatments take 30–60 minutes each, twice a week for three to five weeks, and there is no need to use an anaesthetic or to stay in hospital. There may be some pain in the area of the prostate or bladder, slight bleeding and temporary worsening of obstruction. The preliminary reports show some improvement in symptoms, flow rates and residual urine volumes in the early months after treatment but large scale and long-term studies have not been completed yet.

LASERS Lasers have a reputation for being the most modern, most accurate and most desirable of surgical tools but they have not earned that reputation through prostate surgery. In this field they are still experimental. The size of the channel cut through the prostate by a laser continues to increase for some months after the operation, raising doubts about how accurately the final result can be controlled.

OTHER TECHNIQUES Other techniques such as commissurotomy, prostate incision, dilatation with balloons, ultrasonic treatment and freezing are invented, or more often re-invented, at intervals. Some have been shown not to work reliably, others are unproven; they are all well out of the mainstream of medical practice.

Drug treatment

Drug use, like watchful waiting, is a conservative treatment as the effects are reversible when the drugs are stopped and it does not preclude the use of other treatments afterwards.

Drug treatment always seems the most hopeful area of therapy because there is always the possibility of a new drug being developed, highly effective for a particular disease and with minimal side-effects. In the case of prostate enlargement, this hopeful possibility is exactly that – a hopeful possibility. It has not happened yet.

There are two main groups of drugs in use which can help to relieve the obstruction of an enlarged prostate – alpha-blockers and drugs that affect hormone activity. They are described shortly, along with other less established drug treatments. All these drugs have to be taken indefinitely, they all have side-effects and none is so effective as an operation.

There are also drugs which are aimed not at reducing the degree of obstruction but at reducing the symptoms of urgency, frequency and urge incontinence. These are described on page 61 in the section on treatment for bladder instability.

Alpha-blockers

Roughly speaking, two-thirds of the pressure in the prostatic part of the urethra is produced simply by the bulk of the enlarged prostate and the other third is produced by tension in the muscles. Like other muscles, these are driven by nerves which release chemicals onto receptors on the muscle surface. Different muscles have different types of receptor. The muscle in the prostate works with 'alpha$_1$' receptors so alpha$_1$ blockers such as indoramin and prazosin make it relax, and this reduces the pressure in the urethra. The muscle in the wall of blood vessels works in the same way and the same drugs are sometimes used to treat high blood pressure.

You cannot expect the alpha-blocking drugs to relieve the obstruction completely, of course, because they only counteract the muscle tension and the muscle tension is only a contributor to the obstruction, not its chief cause. They do ease the symptoms and cause small improvements in the flow rate and residual urine volume but no one suggests that they are a cure. They are a help while you wait for more definitive treatment.

Possible side-effects include stuffy nose, dry mouth, lassitude, dizziness and retrograde ejaculation; these would all disappear when you stopped taking the drug. (Retrograde ejaculation is described in more detail on page 48 as a side-effect of surgery.)

Hormonal manipulation

There is a traditional belief that true eunuchs, castrated before puberty, do not develop prostate enlargement. From this, the idea grew that perhaps castration would cure prostate enlargement and a century ago this idea was actually tried out. As well as being notably unpopular with the patients, the results were disappointing. Men would not accept such treatment until their condition was desperate and at that stage the effect on the prostate was too slow to benefit them.

A refinement of the idea is that it is not the testes which matter so much but the testosterone they produce. Doctors have tested this possibility in the last ten years or so by using drugs which either prevent the production of testosterone or block its action – the patients being men who were too unwell for surgery. The results show that, yes, the gland depends on testosterone and that when it is removed or blocked the enlarged prostate shrinks. However, it only shrinks by about 30 per cent and although this does allow the urine to flow more quickly it does very little to reduce the volume of urine left behind in the bladder. The side-effects of these drugs are also unpleasant: impotence is practically universal, and hot flushes common.

The latest idea is that it is not even testosterone itself which affects the prostate but a derivative of it formed in the cells there. Another line of attack, therefore, is to block the conversion of testosterone into this derivative. The hope is that drugs with this action would have far less severe side-effects as they would not reduce testosterone levels throughout the whole body. These drugs are still in the trial stage.

Other drug treatments for benign enlargement

Various other drug treatments have been tried including clofibrate, cholestyramine, candidicin, cimetidine, curbicin, cernilton, beta-sitosterol and assorted plant extracts. Some of these are intended to reduce cholesterol levels, following the observation that cholesterol builds up in an enlarged prostate but not in a normal ageing one. Others are based on traditional homeopathic and folk remedies. So far, none of them has been tested to such an extent and with such success that they are approved for general use in Britain. It is fairly unlikely that your doctor would suggest using any drug other than an alpha-blocker.

I would caution against buying homeopathic or naturopathic medicines such as you might find in a health-food shop. There are two possibilities with these medicines. Either they contain no active ingredient, in which case they are a waste of money, or they do contain active ingredients (of unknown name and in unknown dose), in which case there is the possibility of side-effects and interactions with other medicines you take or other illnesses you have. Certainly none of them will cure you. Even if you can find a way to ameliorate your symptoms, you should take medical advice to make sure that your underlying prostate problem is not progressing to cause irreversible damage.

Treatment by catheter or stent

Catheters and stents are mechanical treatments which place a metal or plastic pipe through the constricted part of the urethra to hold it open either permanently or temporarily while you pee. Catheters have been in use for centuries and the possibility of intermittent catheter use has been studied again recently, with promising results. A permanent catheter is a last resort for long-term treatment, offered when prostate surgery is impossible or unacceptable. Stents are a much more recent invention which may reduce the need for permanent catheters.

Stent

Stents are short stiff tubes which are placed in the urethra where it passes through the prostate, to hold it open despite the pressure from the enlarged gland. Their advantage is that the procedure of putting them in position is relatively simple and it may be possible for you to have this operation even if you are too ill for a prostatectomy. In fact, at present, they are only used for men in this situation as the thinking goes that prostatectomy is an effective and well-established technique so if you are well enough to have it, you are better off with that than with a new and unproven method.

There are two kinds of stents, a temporary spiral type and a permanent mesh type. The advantage of the mesh type is that eventually the skin of the urethra grows over it, leaving it embedded in the wall where it cannot act as a base for bacteria to grow or for scale to form. Before this happens, in the first 4–6 weeks, it can be removed or repositioned quite easily, but afterwards it would take an operation on a par with prostatectomy to do so. Since it is intended to be a permanent solution, the tube is made wide enough to allow instruments to be passed through it to reach the bladder should this ever become necessary.

The temporary type can always be removed because it does not allow the growth of skin over it but, for the same reason, it remains as a foreign body in contact with the urine so it encourages the growth of bacteria, and it can be dislodged. Scale can also form on the spiral, sometimes to such an extent that the passage becomes blocked. It has disadvantages but perhaps less so than an indwelling catheter which would be the usual alternative when surgery is impossible or has to be delayed.

Indwelling catheter

An indwelling catheter is a tube from the bladder to the outside left permanently in place to drain the urine. There are two kinds – urethral and suprapubic. Urethral catheters are inserted through the natural opening of the penis, using a local anaesthetic gel to make it painless. Suprapubic catheters are placed through a nick in the skin of your abdomen just above the pubic hair, after giving a local anaesthetic injection. A urethral catheter is usually the first choice but a suprapubic catheter would be used if the prostate were so large that it was impossible to place a urethral one, or if other problems developed with it.

The urine drains into a bag strapped to your leg or carried in a sporran on a waist belt during the day, and into a larger bag beside your bed at night. You empty the bag at intervals into the toilet. The district nurse or continence adviser would teach you how to manage the taps and bags.

Catheters need changing every so often, usually every 6–12 weeks, because they gradually become covered with deposits which would block them eventually. Generally, it is the continence adviser or district nurse who visits you to deal with catheter changing.

It takes time to get used to having a catheter. At first, you are likely to have an unpleasant feeling of always wanting to empty your bladder (see Chapter 6, page 99). Also, it is almost inevitable that bacteria will use the catheter as a stepping stone to gain entry to your bladder and will continue to grow in the urine. However, they may not cause you any discomfort and even with infected urine you are better off than with retained urine which can affect your kidneys and is itself prone to infection.

Intermittent self-catheterization

Another approach which has some enthusiastic supporters, although it is not in widespread use, is intermittent self-catheterization. If you have reasonable dexterity it is quite easy to learn to insert a catheter yourself, particularly a modern low-friction catheter with a really slippery surface. Then you can use the catheter at regular intervals to ensure that your bladder empties. It hardly takes longer than normal peeing to insert the tube and let the urine flow through it directly into the toilet. Depending on your own circumstances, you may use it every time you use the toilet, at three- or four-hour intervals, or perhaps just once a day to prevent the accumulation of a large volume of retained urine.

You may find this idea more appealing than having a catheter and drainage bag permanently in place. However, if your doctors are unfamiliar with it they are unlikely to suggest it themselves and may feel unable to try it even if you suggest it. The best way forward then would be to find someone else – another doctor or a continence adviser – who is interested in the technique. If someone with experience of self-catheterization agrees that it is feasible in your case, and would be prepared to teach you, it should be possible to persuade your doctor to let you have a try. If you still meet reluctance, ask the reason. What harm could come of it?

Intermittent self-catheterization is not meant to be a sterile technique. You keep the catheter clean, but it will certainly carry bacteria into the bladder. This is not a great problem, though, and intermittent self-catheterization certainly causes less urinary infection than a permanently indwelling catheter. So long as the bladder is emptied regularly its wall will not be overstretched, the blood flow will be normal and the normal mechanisms of resistance to bacteria will have a good chance of dealing with any invaders.

Bladder training

Bladder training (described in detail on page 112) is not actually a treatment for obstruction but it is often effective against the symptoms of urgency, urge incontinence and frequency, and it is very helpful in regaining full bladder control after a prostate operation. It can also be useful before operation but do check with your doctor before embarking on it. It is a conservative treatment in that you can stop it at any time leaving the system intact, so other treatments can be used successfully afterwards.

Treatment of retention

Chronic retention

If urine is being retained at low pressure and causing no serious symptoms it does not need to be treated but in most cases chronic retention does warrant prompt treatment. If obstruction is the cause of the retention, the obstruction itself will have to be treated, most probably by surgery. In the meanwhile, the urine should be drained from the bladder to avoid further stretching of the bladder muscle and possible damage to the kidneys. Drainage is essential if the urine is being retained at high pressures and preventing the kidneys from working properly, so that they can recover somewhat before being faced with the stress of surgery.

Usually, the form of drainage suggested is an indwelling catheter (page 57). In most areas you will have some priority on the waiting list in this situation so you should not have to live with catheter drainage for many months before surgery. If you prefer the idea of intermittent self-catheterization, discuss the possibility with your doctor, specialist or continence adviser. Even if they are not familiar with the technique, they may be willing to put you in touch with someone else who is.

Acute retention

If you are unable to pass urine at all in the usual way, the immediate treatment is to insert a slender catheter into your bladder and drain the urine out that way (see page 57 for more details about the possible types of catheter). However, there is quite a variation from doctor to doctor and hospital to hospital in who will insert the catheter, how and where, and in what they will do for you afterwards.

Some family doctors will send you directly to hospital, either to the accident and emergency department or to the appropriate specialist department, to have a catheter fitted there. Others will come to you at home and insert a catheter themselves. Afterwards, they may send you straight to the hospital department or they may refer you to see the specialist some time later, although you should not have to wait as long for your appointment as someone without retention.

Most doctors use urethral catheters for acute retention but some hospitals favour suprapubic ones (see page 57) because they make it easier to test whether you are able to empty your bladder in the normal way through the penis after treatment. On the other hand, the urethral catheter has the advantage that there is no cut to heal afterwards.

There may be a clear temporary reason for acute retention which has nothing to do with your prostate – for example drugs given in heart failure, or a hernia repair, or some other operation. Once the immediate problem has cleared up it is very unlikely to recur and there is no need for any further treatment.

More often, although some particular event may trigger the episode of acute retention, the underlying cause is longstanding obstruction by an enlarged prostate and it is the prostate which needs treatment for a long-term cure. The appropriate choice is usually surgery, as described above, and you would have priority over patients with less extreme symptoms. If you have been admitted to hospital, you might even go straight on to surgery without leaving again but it is more likely that you will be waiting for some weeks.

Doctors differ in their opinions about whether the catheter

should stay in meanwhile: some drain the urine and remove the catheter immediately; others leave the catheter in place for a day or two and then remove it; others again would leave a catheter with urine draining into a bag on your leg for the whole time until you go for surgery. This is largely a matter of preference as there is no clear evidence that one system is better than the other, so there is room for you to express your preference too. Would you rather live with a catheter or with the worry that you may have another episode of acute retention?

Treatment of bladder instability

The usual approaches to bladder instability are bladder training (see page 74 and Chapter 8, page 112) or drug treatment, or a combination of the two.

The drugs available are moderately effective and may be useful if you have urgency and similar symptoms either without obstruction or after an operation has removed any obstruction. Unfortunately, they are not suitable to use while the urine flow is obstructed. Some of the drugs act directly on the bladder muscle to relax it, while others block the action of the nerves on the bladder muscle in order to inhibit its contractions; they both naturally reduce the bladder's ability to empty itself and this may lead to acute retention. Their side-effects (blurred vision, dry mouth, dizziness, fatigue) occur because they act in other areas of the body as well as the bladder and the nerves controlling the bladder.

Treatment of stricture or bladder-neck obstruction

Urethral stricture (constriction of the urethra, usually by scarring following an injury or severe infection) and obstruction at the bladder neck are usually treated surgically. The procedures are done in a way similar to the typical prostate operation, using a general or spinal anaesthetic and approaching through the penis, but they are less extensive. For stricture, a single incision lengthwise through the constricted part of the urethra allows it to expand to a normal diameter. For bladder-neck obstruction, one or two incisions in the neck of the bladder have the same effect.

Surgical treatment of a stricture opens the urethra effectively, but it cuts through the muscle of the urethral wall and so spoils the closing mechanism in that area. Normally this does not matter because there is spare capacity in the system and so long as another part of the urethra can close firmly you will still be able to hold your urine. However, if you have already had an operation (such as prostatectomy) or an injury which has damaged another section of the closing mechanism, the surgeon would have to be particularly careful to avoid causing incontinence. Make sure that he is aware of any treatments or injuries you have had before.

Another treatment for urethral stricture is to stretch it by passing a tube or dilator through. Some men suffer repeatedly from strictures and in this case you may be offered the opportunity of intermittent self-catheterization, not to drain urine but to ensure that the urethra remains stretched following an operation.

Treatment of urinary tract infection and prostatitis

Infections are treated with antibiotics. It is preferable to take a urine sample, grow the bacteria from it and check which antibiotics will kill them before choosing the drug, but a doctor may sometimes prescribe first and check afterwards if the symptoms of infection are particularly troublesome.

Antibiotic treatment is usually effective against infections based in the bladder, although these may recur if there is an underlying cause (stones, perhaps, or residual urine) which has not been treated. Infections based in the prostate – one possible cause of prostatitis – are more resistant. The bacteria penetrate into all the tiny crevices of the gland and it is hard to get a high enough dose of drug into position to overcome them. Treatment works best when there is a single sudden episode of infection; if infection is long-standing, and especially if the bacteria have colonized tiny stones in the prostate, a cure cannot be guaranteed.

Prostatectomy is a treatment of desperation for prostatitis. It helps occasionally but since the gland cannot be removed completely it is likely that infection, or whatever the cause is, will remain in the remaining tissue.

Recurrent perineal pain (pain in the 'saddle' area) does not necessarily mean that you have prostatitis. There may be no significant medical reason for it at all. With no clear cause, there is no clear cure although you may get some help from treatment aimed directly at the symptoms, e.g. painkillers. Sometimes it is better to concentrate your efforts on living with the condition rather than attempting to cure it, understanding that it is an annoyance but not a sign of serious illness.

Treatment of stones

Very large stones have to be removed surgically through a cut in the abdomen. Smaller ones can be made to disintegrate by mechanical or ultrasonic means using instruments passed through the urethra, or by the use of focused shock waves from outside the body. The fragments pass out through the urethra later with the urine.

Treatment of cancer

Prostate cancers vary enormously. Some are so torpid that they are never going to grow large enough or spread far enough to do you any damage in your natural lifetime. Others are dangerously invasive. It is essential to know as much as you can about the cancer before trying to make any decision about treatment.

Doctors tell the grade of a cancer, which gives a good prediction of its potential for harm, by looking at it under the microscope. Low-grade cancers look almost like normal prostate gland, and they behave almost like normal prostate gland. High-grade, dangerous, cancers look quite different because the cells are too busy multiplying to bother showing any special prostate features. It is also important to know the stage of the cancer, that is, how far it has spread already.

It is quite common to find cancer cells incidentally when the prostate is removed for benign enlargement. This happens in about one case in eight. Usually, the cancer is very small and the cells are only slightly abnormal, so it can be quite sensible to do nothing more than keep an eye on the situation. Often, no further development occurs and no further action is ever needed. The exception to this course of non-treatment might be for a young man because the cancer would then have a longer time in which to develop and cause trouble. Active treatment might also be appropriate if the cells had a higher grade of abnormality.

At the other extreme are high-grade cancers which have already escaped from the prostate and established colonies in other organs of the body such as the lymph nodes and bones. There is little treatment for these late-stage cancers that can prolong life, and treatment therefore has to be aimed at relieving pain and other symptoms.

Between the two extremes are cancers which can and should be treated, and there are four main planks to treatment: surgery, radiation, hormonal manipulation and chemotherapy. The first two are most appropriate when the cancer is still contained within the prostate, the last two if it has spread beyond the gland itself.

The treatments are described extremely briefly here. If you are in this situation, your doctors should describe the exact treatments they are suggesting, their likely success and side-effects, and the reasons for choosing them in your own particular case. You may also find useful information in books about cancer.

Surgery

The surgical treatment for prostate cancer is radical prostatectomy in which the prostate is removed along with its associated lymph nodes and some surrounding tissue. It is done through an incision low in the abdomen. In the past, radical prostatectomy routinely caused impotence by damaging the nerves supplying the blood vessels of the penis, but there is a new version of the operation which spares those nerves and makes it quite likely that you will still be able to have erections afterwards.

Radical prostatectomy is fairly effective so long as the cancer is confined to the prostate but it is more or less useless if the cancer has spread to other organs, so you should expect to have extensive tests beforehand to make sure that there are no cancer cells anywhere else in the body.

Radiation

Radiation kills cells and it kills cancer cells more easily than normal ones because cells which are multiplying fast are more sensitive than others. The main problem is that radiation does also cause some damage to normal cells and this limits the dose which can be given. The more accurately the radiation can be aimed the better, as this allows the highest dose possible to reach the malignant cells without causing undue harm to normal tissue. The radiation can be directed at the prostate from a machine outside the body or tiny pieces of radioactive material can be implanted right inside the prostate as a close range source of radiation.

If the cancer has spread into other parts of the body it may be helpful to have whole body radiation but this is likely to have side-effects as it is impossible to avoid other sensitive cells such as the bone marrow and gut.

Hormonal manipulation

Prostate cancer cells retain some signs of their ancestry and remain like normal prostate cells in depending on the male hormone testosterone. By removing testosterone, their growth is slowed or stopped. The most obvious way of reducing the level of testosterone is to remove the testicles surgically, but there are often psychological difficulties and many men and many surgeons are understandably reluctant to do it. It is possible to achieve the same effect with drugs and these have now been formulated in such a way that you can take them by injection once a month instead of having to swallow pills every day. There is a little more information about these drugs on page 55 because they have also been investigated, less successfully, for use in benign enlargement of the prostate.

Hormonal treatment can give you respite for a long time but sadly it is not a total cure. Eventually a variant cancer emerges which can manage without testosterone, leaving radiation and chemotherapy as the remaining options for treatment.

Chemotherapy

Chemotherapy is used in the same way for prostate cancers as for others, and with the same side-effects. Like radiation, the drugs kill cancer cells selectively because they are multiplying faster than normal cells but it also harms normal tissues including the bone marrow, gut and skin, and there is no way yet of targeting the drug specifically to the cancer. Nausea and vomiting have always been particularly unpleasant side-effects of chemotherapy but new anti-emetic drugs are helping to limit these difficulties.

6

Waiting for Surgery

How long will the wait be?

The picture over the whole country

Department of Health figures for the whole country at the time of writing show nearly twenty thousand men waiting for prostatectomy. About one in six of them have already been waiting for six months or more, and about one in fourteen have already waited for a year or more. On the other hand, of those men who had actually had their operations in the six-month period recorded, half had been treated within two months of going onto a list and the average wait had been about four months. The figures show that a substantial proportion of men are treated quickly, within weeks of a consultant deciding that treatment is needed, but that those who wait longer often wait a very great deal longer.

It is almost pointless to try to guess what wait you will have by looking at national or even regional figures. The figures disguise differences between individual consultants and hospitals, and even if you knew the length of individual lists you could not predict your likely wait unless you knew what sort of patients made them up. Treatment policy, on the whole, is to take people off the waiting list according to medical priority, not according to length of wait. If you are a case of middling priority, you would do equally well (or badly) on a short list of mostly urgent cases or a long list of mostly non-urgent cases.

You should be treated quickly if your medical need is urgent, for example, if your kidneys are showing signs of injury as a result of the obstruction. Most surgeons would also consider it significant if your bladder was failing to empty completely so that you were constantly retaining a large volume of urine, or if you had ever had an episode of acute retention – complete inability to pee – following on from prostate enlargement. If there was no sign of any serious medical consequences, you would be given a lower priority however annoying your symptoms were. In the lower priority group you could find yourself facing a long and uncertain wait, your own treatment constantly delayed in favour of new patients with more immediate needs.

The picture for your own particular case

The best way to find out how long you are likely to have to wait is simply to ask. Your consultant should be able to give you a fairly accurate estimate, knowing the number of patients on his or her waiting list and the urgency of your situation compared with theirs.

There are other points you may want to check about the waiting list, such as making sure that you would not lose your place if you were unable to attend on the first date offered because of a funeral, family wedding, holiday or similar event at the time or shortly afterwards (some consultants like you to stay in the area for six weeks after the operation; check whether yours thinks this is necessary). You could also ask how much notice you will be given when a date is arranged for your operation, and whether there is a standby scheme to fill the vacancies created by late cancellations. The best person to approach with questions of this sort is the person who actually manages the list; the consultant can tell you who this is.

What can I do to make the wait shorter?

Shortening the wait on the NHS

One very simple way to reduce the wait is to be prepared to go into hospital at short notice, and make sure that the waiting list manager has you on the list of standby patients. But this may not help much if you are classed, medically, as a low priority as there will often be higher priority people above you on the list who are also willing to go in at short notice.

Make sure that your doctor knows of, and informs the consultant of, any special circumstances which might influence their assessment of your priority – for example, if your condition is making it impossible to carry out your business or job, or care for a dependent relative. Also make sure they know if your condition worsens – this may shunt you up the queue too.

Consider the possibility of transferring to a different list; some areas, some hospitals and some consultants have shorter waiting lists than others. Your doctor will have some information about the waiting times in your own area, and the College of Health operates a National Waiting List Helpline with constantly updated information to help patients and doctors find the hospitals with the shortest waiting times for each speciality (Tel: 081 983 1133, Monday to Friday 10 a.m. to 4 p.m.).

You need to find out the waiting times for outpatient appointments as well as for surgery. These figures are not collected nationally so the best sources of information are the Community Health Councils and the hospitals themselves, where you can ask to speak to the secretary of one of the consultants in urology (or general surgery if there is no urology department). The telephone numbers are available in the *Yellow Pages* as well as in various medical directories and hospital yearbooks available in libraries.

However, although it is relatively simple to locate a shorter list, it is much less straightforward to have yourself referred onto it. First of all, your own doctor must be amenable and there are many possible objections. He will probably be worried about sending you to a surgeon he does not know personally, and he may wonder whether the shortness of the surgeon's list is because other doctors who do know him have a poor opinion of his work. There is a question of whether a local surgeon would be prepared to do follow-up treatment if there were complications following an operation done in another district. There may be difficulties with the practice budget, with the district health authority's rules, or with the procedures to follow when referring outside the usual contractual arrangements.

You will also need to take account of the extra waits that a new referral will bring with it. It may be some time before a district health authority will even decide whether to allow the referral, and you will have to wait for an outpatient appointment as well before the new consultant can consider putting you on a list for surgery.

Going private

Assuming that you have no moral objections to private treatment, probably the first question to ask is 'What will it cost?' and the answer is that it varies enormously. A very rough guide, at 1992 prices, would be at least two thousand pounds, more probably three thousand, and more still in London.

If you are considering going private, it is important to find out exactly what is included in the price. Many private hospitals quote a fixed price but without including the fees for the surgeon and anaesthetist. Others quote a fixed price including the surgeon's and anaesthetist's fees but not including the outpatient appointments you will need. Others again charge per day of hospital stay, so you cannot predict the cost at the outset with any accuracy at all. Check whether the price includes consultants' fees, outpatient visits, investigations such as x-rays, drugs, dressings, follow-up checks and additional treatment if the first operation is unsuccessful or has complications – and check how much these items are likely to cost. Ask about the facilities in the hospital concerned, both the hotel amenities and the medical facilities such as availability of intensive care and 24-hour medical cover.

It is important, if you have private health insurance, to find out exactly what it covers. Not all insurances cover all aspects of all treatments, and some are tied to particular hospitals.

The route into private treatment is via your family doctor who can refer you to a consultant as a private patient. You can choose the consultant and/or the hospital, taking account of your information on cost and facilities and any limitations on your insurance, or your doctor can advise you.

Am I likely to get worse while waiting?

General progression of symptoms

Once your prostate is enlarged, it is not going to shrink again so do not hope for a miracle remission which will make your operation unnecessary. In fact, when measuring the rate of urine flow, the volume of urine left in the bladder and other objective features, it is clear that the disease does gradually progress. A half to three-quarters of men get worse over three to five years, although up to a quarter actually improve a little. However, you are not expecting to wait anything like so long as three years, so you should expect little real change before your operation.

As for your symptoms, though, those are much more variable and you will notice ups and downs from week to week because the symptoms do not depend simply on the size of your prostate. The few studies available on this question of how the symptoms develop suggest that, over three to five years, between a quarter and a half of men will feel that they have improved and a similar proportion will feel that they have got worse. There is some evidence that if you are going to get worse you will do so slowly, whereas if you are going to get better you will do so relatively quickly – in less than six months.

Major complications such as kidney failure and serious urinary infection are rare in patients who are waiting for treatment – so rare that they do not show up in the studies mentioned above. If there is any reason to think your kidneys are being affected, you should have priority on the waiting list in any case and be treated with little delay.

Acute retention

A sudden complete inability to pee is the one serious complication which is fairly common, but it is very difficult indeed to work out how likely it is to happen to you or to anybody else on the waiting list. Quite a proportion of men (10–40 per cent) do not go to their doctors at all until they have an attack of retention. If prostate enlargement caused that first attack it is very likely to cause a repeat episode in the following weeks or months. Among men who have not previously had acute retention, the estimates for how many will have an attack within five years vary from 4 to 50 per cent! Since you expect to be waiting a much shorter time than five years, however, your chance of suffering an episode of acute retention is much less than this.

It is also very difficult to predict which particular people will be unlucky. The only clue is that men who have a very hesitant start to their peeing, and especially those who have worse hesitancy when their bladders are full, are more likely to suffer than others. If this applies to you, avoid holding on for any length of time after you first feel a need to empty your bladder. It is also wise to avoid other potential triggers such as substantial amounts of alcohol and undue cold or stress.

Try not to panic when you first think that you cannot pee. Nobody can pee while they panic. Leave it for half an hour or so and try again. If that does not work, run yourself a warm bath, get in, lie down, relax and try emptying your bladder there. The warmth relaxes the muscles and the pressures are distributed differently when you are in water. It can work. If not, call your doctor for help.

Your general health

Look after your general health as much as you can so that when you do finally go for surgery you are in the best possible shape; it will make a tremendous difference to how well you recover afterwards. Fresh fruit, vegetables and protein are as important as ever in your diet, and if you eat plenty of fruit, vegetables and brown bread or wholemeal cereals you will naturally be eating enough fibre. This will help to prevent constipation which would put extra pressure on your prostate and possibly make your symptoms worse.

70

A certain amount of exercise is still good for you. Take account of your general condition and any particular health problems you have, but be as active as you can within your own limitations.

An enlarged prostate is no reason to give up sexual activity. Sex will not make your symptoms worse and it will not harm your partner. It may actually make you feel better.

No doubt you are tired of people nagging you to give up smoking but it is worth doing if you can as you will take the anaesthetic better if your lungs are clear. A novel product has been introduced fairly recently which your doctor can prescribe to help you. It is nicotine plasters like ordinary sticking plasters. The nicotine is absorbed through your skin so you can deal with giving up smoking first without the more difficult problem of giving up nicotine.

Managing the symptoms while waiting

Drinking

It is natural to feel that you would have less trouble if you produced less urine but in fact it is a big mistake to cut down on your fluid intake. You should be having three to four pints of watery drinks each day, that is, six large mugs or ten cups.

If you drink too little your urine will be very concentrated because your body still has to get rid of the same quantity of waste chemicals as always; they will just be dissolved in a smaller amount of water. Concentrated urine itself tends to give you a sense of urgency because it irritates the bladder and the urethra so this is no help in overcoming the problem. Also, if you drink very little you are making it difficult for your kidneys to do their job of removing waste materials from the body. There is a limit to how concentrated they can make the urine. If you make the urine volume too small, it may be impossible to dissolve all the waste that should be removed and it is harmful to have it remaining in your bloodstream.

A third point against cutting down the amount you drink is that it makes you vulnerable to bladder infections. You are already more than usually vulnerable if your bladder is not emptying completely because the remaining pool of urine is an ideal breeding ground for bacteria. The best defence against urinary infection is a constant flow of fresh dilute urine to wash bacteria out of the bladder before they have much chance to multiply.

There is some sense in restricting your drinking before a special event, like a visit to the theatre where you will particularly want to avoid frequent toilet visits, or in the evening if you are very much disturbed by waking to empty your bladder at night. However, it is essential to drink plenty at other times so that your daily intake is sufficient. Remember that there is a lag between drinking and urine production, and it takes about three hours after stopping drinking before urine production slows right down, so you would need to plan ahead.

Alcoholic and caffeine-containing drinks both promote urine production to a greater extent than plain liquids but this is not a problem so long as you drink enough fluid to cater for the increased production. Caffeine is also a stimulant which makes bladder control more precarious. It is worth avoiding tea, coffee and cola drinks for the few hours before bedtime and special occasions.

Try to spread your drinking fairly evenly through the day to avoid sudden large changes in the urine flow to the bladder. An abrupt surge in urine production may well cause urgency and it is just possible, if you were on the borderline for an attack of acute retention, that this could be the final provocation which brought it on.

Peeing

Problems of hesitancy and slow stream

The chief piece of advice in this section is simple to give and hard to follow: be patient. There is a limited amount you can do for yourself to make urinating easier, but you can at least avoid making it harder for yourself. If you try to hurry and get tense and frustrated, the muscles around the urethra will tense up too, constrict the pipe and inhibit the workings of your bladder into the bargain. Having a naturally patient nature is a bonus in this situation, but it is not essential. Anyone can learn techniques of relaxation (see page 81), and you can put your mind to overcoming your exasperation in other ways too, at least for long enough to pee in peace.

Yes, peeing takes longer than it used to and that is irritating, but try working out exactly how much longer it takes. A minute each time? Two minutes? How much is that in a day, really? And what did you want to do with that time? Think about making time spent in the toilet less dull. Put a magazine there, or the sort of book you can dip into, or the radio, or some simple job that you can do little by little.

It is worth having a try at peeing sitting down, too. It will probably feel odd at first, but if you can get used to it you may find that your bladder empties more readily. It is often easier to relax when sitting, and it frees your hands for reading or doing something else to take your mind off the rather tiresome process of peeing. Sitting is also a useful ruse to escape from public situations where difficulty in getting started is a real embarrassment, like half-time at a football match with a rowdy queue behind you. No one knows that you have gone into a cubicle for a sit-down pee . . .

If delay in getting the stream started is a problem for you, try the old trick of running a tap. It is simple, but it can help.

Problems of frequency and urgency

There are two likely causes for frequent or urgent need to empty your bladder when you have an enlarged prostate. One is that your bladder is not emptying completely during peeing: with urine remaining in the bladder, you only have to produce a small volume more before the bladder is burstingly full again and needs to be emptied. The other is that your bladder has become unstable as a result of the obstruction, or perhaps it was unstable beforehand. Unstable bladders overreact to moderate volumes of urine and provoke an overwhelming sense of need to pee.

Either way, you should do what you can to help your bladder to empty completely when you do go to the toilet. Use the tips suggested above for hesitancy and slow stream, and see if 'double voiding' is any help. Double voiding just means peeing once, waiting a few minutes to let the bladder muscle recover from the exertion and peeing again. It may be that the bladder fails to empty completely the first time simply because it tires from the strain of expelling urine through the constriction. It may also be that it was working at a disadvantage the first time because the bladder was overfull; like other muscles, the bladder works most efficiently when it is in the middle of its range of stretch.

Holding out against the sensation of urgent need to urinate, at least for long enough to reach the toilet in comfort, is another skill. It is easier to manage it sitting than standing, and easier standing still than walking. Cross your legs if it helps, tense up your pelvic floor (see page 114), breathe slowly and regularly (see page 81) and think of something else (see page 113). Once the first intensity of need has passed, set off for the lavatory cautiously and be

73

prepared to stop again on the way if need be to overcome any further feelings of urgency.

BLADDER TRAINING Bladder training uses all the tricks of holding on mentioned above in a deliberate, methodical way. The idea is very simple: you keep a record of the times when you pee, and the amounts, and very gradually, over weeks or months, increase the intervals until, ideally, you can manage three or four hours between visits to the toilet and produce a volume of a half to three-quarters of a pint (300–400 ml) at a time.

Bladder training is the recognized way of dealing with bladder instability, frequency and urgency where there is no apparent physical cause for the problem. It is very appropriate to use the technique after your operation to retrain your bladder into normal behaviour and it is described in detail in the chapter on recovery from surgery (see Chapter 8, page 112). It may be helpful to use bladder training before surgery if instability is the main reason for your frequency and urgency, but probably not if the root of the trouble is your bladder's failure to empty completely – and certainly not if you find that holding on makes it particularly difficult to get the flow started when you do reach the lavatory. Consult your doctor and specialist first.

Dealing with dribbles

A dribbly finish to urination is one of the symptoms of the obstruction and it is one of those things which cannot be changed before surgery, to be accepted with serenity if you can manage it.

However, small dribbles of urine which wet your pants a few moments *after* you have finished peeing can be prevented. These are not uncommon, and medically speaking they are usually not significant, but they can be embarrassing. The cause is urine left in the U-bend of the urethra at the end of urination which dribbles out when the lower sphincter relaxes a few minutes later. With a large prostate obstructing the way, the system cannot squeeze this back into the bladder automatically as it normally would, so you need to move the urine into the penis instead. Then it can be removed by shaking or squeezing as usual. Press upwards on the skin a little way forward of the anus and keep the upward pressure while you draw your fingers forward to the base of your scrotum.

You should not expect any dribbling of urine at other times. If you do have any, mention it to your doctor so that some action can be taken.

Night-time peeing

The disturbance to your sleep caused by having to get up to pee in the night can be an enormous nuisance, and it is exacerbated by the fact that as you get older you sleep more lightly, wake more easily and find it more difficult to get back to sleep again. On the other hand, you actually need less sleep than you used to so, although you may not like being awake in the dark and lonely hours, it is probably not doing you any particular harm. Night-time sleep is no more valuable than daytime naps and it is a matter of preference whether you use naps to make up for lost sleep or avoid them to increase your chances of sleeping through the night.

The advice about drinking on page 71 can help to reduce urine production and cut down the number of times you need to get up at night, perhaps from three or four to one or two. It is not a complete solution but if it strikes you as an improvement worth trying for, drink sparingly in the three or four hours before bedtime and especially avoid tea, coffee, chocolate and alcoholic drinks at this time. Do remember to drink plenty during the daytime to make up, though.

To help with getting back to sleep afterwards, keep your bed cosy and warm with an extra blanket, or even an electric blanket. Keep yourself warm while you visit the toilet, too, to avoid becoming too widely awake, and if you can avoid a long hike to the lavatory and bright lights on the way, so much the better. Chamber pots may be unfashionable, but they have their uses. Deliberate relaxation (see page 81) is as good as a sleeping pill once you get back to bed.

If you really cannot get back to sleep, try not to fret over it too much. The chances are that you just do not need to sleep so much, and if the need to pee had not woken you something else would have done. You can pass the time with reading, or with the radio (the BBC World Service broadcasts throughout the night), or with tapes of music, stories or plays. Use earphones if you are concerned about disturbing your partner.

The use of medicines

There are a few drugs which can help with the symptoms of prostate enlargement but, like all drugs, they have side-effects, so doctors tend to avoid them unless your symptoms are particularly severe (they are described on pages 54 and 61). Many other drugs given for all sorts of conditions have side-effects which could make your urinary symptoms worse. Carry on taking them unless your doctor advises differently but do remind him that you have an enlarged prostate when he is considering prescribing any drugs for you, whether they are for an ongoing condition like a heart problem or for something short term, and tell him if any new medicine seems to make your symptoms worse.

It is also a good idea to mention your prostate problem to the pharmacist when you go to collect a prescription. Pharmacists are specialists in drugs and their interactions, and although they cannot change the prescription they can mention it to the doctor if they spot any potential problems that he has missed. It is an especially good idea to discuss with the pharmacist if you are buying any medicines over the counter without a prescription, such as treatment for coughs, colds or hayfever. These too can contain drugs which it may be wiser for you to avoid.

Avoiding cold and stress

You only need to look back to some particularly important and nerve-racking occasion to recognize the disruptive effect of emotional stress on your bladder control. Cold also makes matters worse because it is a physical stress which activates the sympathetic division of your nervous system, the one which is linked with the action hormone adrenalin. It manages, paradoxically, to make both urgency and hesitancy worse at the same time.

Managing the strain of waiting

There is no question that the symptoms of prostate enlargement are exasperating, and that it is a strain to be faced with an uncertain wait for treatment. You may well feel frustrated, or irritated, or resentful or depressed. You may hate the apparent loss of control caused by the urgency of your urinary needs, or be embarrassed to go out in public or be afraid of how much worse the situation is going to get. You may find that the prostate problem brings other difficult questions into your mind that you would have preferred to ignore – reminding you in an inescapable way that you are getting older, for example.

Identify the real problem

With each aspect of the situation that bothers you, ask yourself honestly what the problem really is. You dislike having to go to the toilet so often. Why? Is it because it interrupts your work, or because it is painful to walk to the toilet with an arthritic knee, or because the toilet is cold and uncomfortable, or because it makes you feel helpless? So what? Is the interruption really affecting your work by disrupting a meeting or forcing you to park your lorry on the hard shoulder, for instance, or is it really just a minor nuisance?

Carry on interrogating yourself with a succession of Why?s and So-what?s, just as a small child would do, and go on beyond the point where the answer seems so obvious that you cannot think of the words for it. Often that is exactly the point where you will find one reason sheltering behind another, your unconscious using the prostate problem as a scapegoat for quite unrelated concerns. It is important to chase these worries out and try to deal with them yourself; you cannot expect the prostate operation to solve unconnected problems.

Once you have worked out what is really distressing you, you are in a much better position to do something about it. Not all problems can be solved at root, but you can minimize the impact of most of them by planning and taking simple practical steps.

Even if it turns out that your anxieties have less to do with your prostate than you first thought, you can approach them in the same way. Look at the practical impact of whatever it is, and look for practical ways to lessen it. And try looking at the 'problem' from a different direction; you may be able to see it as an opportunity. The loss of a working routine on retirement is also the freedom to decide for yourself how to spend your day, and whilst growing older inevitably brings some loss of physical abilities it also brings a lifetime's memories, a lifetime's experience and perhaps a wiser, more philosophical viewpoint.

Take control

The basic problem is a problem in your urinary system which is causing various difficulties. It is not you yourself who is a problem or a nuisance or weak. Look at the problem as something separate from yourself, split it into smaller problems and take control of them. You have already started this process by thinking of ways to reduce the impact of some of the symptoms.

Use information, planning and practical measures to keep the problem in its place, and you in control.

Inform yourself

Information is the best antidote to anxiety because uncertainty is very unsettling in itself and, besides, it usually turns out that reality is nothing like as alarming as your worst imaginings.

For fears about the operation itself, read Chapter 7, and talk to your own doctor and surgeon about what to expect. If you are afraid that you may suddenly be unable to pee at all, talk to your doctor and find out what you need to know in addition to the information on pages 60 (Chapter 5) and 70. How quickly would he be able to come and what should you say to the receptionist to make sure you are taken seriously? Would he advise you to take yourself straight to the accident and emergency department of the local hospital instead? How would you get there?

You should be able to go away on holidays and visits without worrying that you may lose your place on the waiting list if you are called up for operation while you are away. Find out about the workings of the hospital waiting list and the system of call-up to reassure yourself on this point.

If you are worried about how your household will manage without you, find out what help is available from various sources. Family and neighbours are often happy to look after houses, plants and pets, and social services and voluntary organizations can give support for more serious responsibilities such as looking after a disabled relative. Your local council office, library, Citizens Advice Bureau or doctor can help you to find the right person to contact in order to make suitable arrangements.

Find out about any forms that need filling in in connection with your work, your pension, your private health insurance and anything else that could conceivably be affected by a hospital stay.

Make plans

Planning follows on from getting information. Once you know what your doctor would do if, for example, you had a sudden retention of urine, you can plan what you would do if the worst came to the worst. That does not stop it happening, but it takes a lot of the worry out of it.

It is a good idea to plan ahead for your hospital stay, particularly if you have told the hospital that you can go in at short notice. Think

78

of the things to be cancelled (milk, newspapers, social commitments). Think of the things to be looked after (the house by a neighbour if it is empty, perhaps, and the dog by a family member). Think of the people to be informed (family, social clubs, work), and the items to take to hospital with you (see Chapter 8). Think of the arrangements for you – and later your visitors – to reach hospital. If your home will be empty, plan to clear out the fridge before you go, switch off the water and possibly the central heating (this may be better left on low in winter to avoid dampness and freezing pipes), secure all the windows, lock all the doors and *take your key with you.*

Remember that you will not feel wonderfully well for several weeks after the operation so some jobs, Christmas shopping for instance, may be best done beforehand in order to leave a time clear for your convalescence afterwards.

Take practical steps

Some general practical points are covered in the section on managing your symptoms (see page 71). Beyond that, it is a question of identifying the things that bother *you* particularly and using your ingenuity to overcome them. For a simple example, if you like to go to the cinema, choose an aisle seat so that you can get out to the toilets without disturbing a whole row of people.

Talk it over

Talk to your partner

It is obvious, but easily overlooked, that your bladder problem is not yours alone. Your partner needs to know what to expect almost as much as you do. She will be very aware of your symptoms, she will be concerned about how they may develop, she will care what is going to happen to you in hospital. And in social situations, she will be the one left facing the rest of your friends and wondering what to say when you disappear into the toilets for the fourth time in the evening.

Talk to your friends

I am not suggesting that you should blurt your private medical details to all and sundry, but your close friends will certainly notice if you are out for a pee every hour and they will be less concerned – and you will be less embarrassed – if you can give them some idea of the reason for it. If you keep totally silent on the subject, they may even wonder whether you have realized that anything is wrong, and worry about how they can point out to you, tactfully, that perhaps you should see a doctor. You will find your own way to be as vague or precise, serious or humorous as you want to be. Just saying 'There I go again' as you set off to the toilet for the third time at least lets them know that you are aware of it, and something along the lines of 'Yes, the waterworks are playing up a bit. Still, I've got the plumbers coming in before too long' covers the main points quite succinctly.

People are much more tolerant than you think, especially if you take them into your confidence. They are not likely to regard you as a nuisance when they understand the situation. Perhaps you are reluctant to ask to use someone else's toilet, feeling it to be rude, but would you think it a rude request from a friend in the same situation? Maybe it is time to drop this particular rule of politeness altogether, for the convenience of all.

Talk to yourself

Yes, really, talking to yourself is a good way to deal with some situations. Maybe you feel that the young men in the pub are noticing your constant visits to the toilets and laughing at you. They are not, of course. They are much too busy with their own concerns and conversations. They probably have not even noticed you. Did you ever notice other men going to the toilets when you were in your twenties? It can help to overcome your embarrassment if you simply repeat it over to yourself as you walk past, 'They're not interested in me, they're not counting, they've got their own concerns'. Do you care very much what they think anyway? They are young and ignorant, and their turn will come soon enough.

Keep up your social contacts

Do not let your bladder push you into dropping your regular social activities, whatever they are. Your friends and interests are much too important to lose because of your temporary urinary difficulties. It would be depressing to stay at home on your own with no one but your family for company even just for the time until your operation, but in practice it can be so difficult to start again with going to your club, your bowls match, your card games or whatever after six months or a year away that you can find you have dropped out of them permanently almost by accident.

If you find it really impossible to keep up with your old activities, at least look for some other way of keeping up with your old friends.

Relaxation

Relaxation is a skill. It is not a difficult skill but you will definitely get better at it the more you practise. There are two basic techniques: breathing and muscle-clenching.

Practise the breathing, at first, sitting comfortably with your eyes shut. Later you can do it wherever you need to and in any position. Breathe normally and settle down. Now watch and feel the air as it goes into your body, tracking it through your nostrils, down your throat and deep into your lungs, carrying fresh energy with it. Let the breath out, carrying tiredness and tension with it. As you carry on doing this, you will find that you are naturally breathing more slowly and deeply. Concentrate wholly on the breathing, and keep going for five minutes or as much longer as you like. When you have practised regularly for some time, you will find that you can calm yourself in an instant in tricky situations by going straight into this slow, regular, deliberate way of breathing.

Muscle-clenching is best learnt lying down in a comfortable position. Starting with your hands, clench them up tightly for a few seconds, then let them relax. Move on to your arms and shoulders, then go down to your feet and work back up your legs and body bit by bit. Each time, tense the muscles up for a few seconds and then, as you breathe out, let them flop. Concentrate particularly on the muscles around your shoulders, the back of your neck, and in your face, raising your eyebrows as high as you can, and opening your mouth as wide as you can, before you let them relax. When you have worked over your whole body, you should be perfectly relaxed – although to begin with you will probably find tension creeping back into your hands while you relax your neck, for instance.

As you practise, you will become more aware of tension in your body at other times and you will be able to let it go more easily, often without even needing to clench deliberately beforehand. Combining deliberate muscle relaxation with breathing gives you a really powerful method of overcoming tension in all sorts of situations.

That was a very brief outline. It is much better to learn from a live teacher. If you are interested, look for a class run by your health centre or local education authority, either in relaxation or in yoga or one of the other meditative traditions which use similar breathing exercises.

A *last word*

You have lived through lots of phases in your life, and this is just another one. It will not go on for ever. In a year or so, when you can look back, you will find plenty to laugh about. In the meantime, just remember that your bladder is not your boss.

7

Your Hospital Stay

Going into hospital

Contact with the hospital

Unless you have said that you are available at short notice – in which case you might be telephoned one day for admission to hospital the next – you should receive a letter a few weeks before the date planned for your operation. Read it very carefully; it ought to explain exactly what to do and whom to contact with any queries. If you cannot go in at the time arranged, contact the hospital straight away and explain the problem. You should not lose your place on the waiting list. You will probably be asked to contact the hospital in any case to confirm that you have received the letter and intend to accept the offer of treatment.

You may also be asked to telephone the ward shortly before your planned admission to check that your bed is still available, and it would be wise to do so whether or not you are asked. If several beds have had to be used for emergencies, making your planned operation impossible this week, the way to find out is the day before on the telephone, not after you have starved since midnight and driven two hours to reach the place.

If you are unwell, with a heavy cold or 'flu, for example, shortly before you expect to go into hospital, contact the ward or your own doctor for advice. It may not be safe to operate if you are ill, and it is better for everybody to know in good time. Then another patient can be called up to use the bed, another time can be arranged for your operation, and you do not waste your time on a pointless journey to hospital.

Even if information is missing from the letter, it is not difficult to find out. Phone the hospital and ask to speak to your consultant's secretary, or to the admissions office. They will know the name of the relevant ward, the name of the nurse in charge of it, the name of the person in charge of admissions to it – or they will know someone who does. Explain what your question is about, ask who is the best person to talk to, and be prepared to follow a chain of several people before you get your answer.

The hospital may ask you to come in the day before your

operation, or early on the actual day of operation. In this case, you need to starve yourself for twelve hours beforehand (see page 86).

Arrangements for your home

I mentioned the main points about looking after your home in Chapter 6 and ideally you will have thought about your plans before receiving your admission letter. If neighbours are helping by keeping an eye on your home, feeding your cat, watering your plants or whatever, it is a good idea to take their telephone numbers into hospital with you, and to give them the number of the hospital and the name of your ward.

What to take with you

You need pyjamas, slippers and a dressing gown to wear. After the operation you can perfectly well wear light clothes if you prefer, but pyjamas are very practical during the numerous medical examinations beforehand, and you will need them for night-time anyway. You do not need much spare clothing for a short stay but it is worth having spare underpants and pyjamas in case of mishaps after the operation while your urinary system is unsettled.

Remember your towel, razor, comb and personal washing things – soap, flannel, toothbrush, denture cleaner and so on.

Take enough to do, too. It is hard to concentrate on anything very demanding with doctors examining you, nurses taking your temperature, other patients' visitors talking and with being tired out from your operation but you will soon be looking for ways to pass your time. There will probably be a dayroom with a television which you can use when you are up and about again, although the other patients' preference for channel may not match yours. Think of books (and reading glasses if you need them), letters to write, a radio (or portable TV, or tape recorder) with headphones. Remember to put in new batteries or take spares.

It is comforting to have some food of your own such as fruit, which you can eat when you choose and not at fixed hospital mealtimes, and it is a good idea to take in some fruit squash or juice to flavour the jugfulls of water you will be expected to drink.

Check whether you should take any forms, allowance books or certificates to do with your pension, social security, health insurance or employment with you. You may need to use them or to have them signed by the hospital.

Take the bottles of any medicines that you normally use with just a few pills in, enough for a day or two, and make sure that the ward staff know what they are and what they are for. There is no point taking large quantities as the hospital will give you the same medicines from its own pharmacy, not from your bottles, and you may not get them back.

A small amount of money is useful for the telephone and for small items such as newspapers from the hospital shop or trolley. You should also budget enough money for the journey home at the end of your stay.

Avoid taking valuable things, including large amounts of money, credit cards, jewellery. There is no use for them in hospital, they are at risk of being stolen on the ward (the lockers do not lock) and it is a nuisance to have them put away in the hospital safe – and even more of a nuisance to get them taken out again, particularly outside office hours when no one has access to it.

The ward staff will also be happier if you leave your mobile phone at home. It can interfere with the hospital bleep system, and it can annoy your fellow patients a great deal. You should have easy access to a payphone in or near the ward, most likely one which can be wheeled around and plugged in by your bed.

Visitors

Your admission letter should tell you what are the preferred visiting hours on the ward so that you can tell potential visitors before you leave home. If not, you can find out by telephone or when you first go in. Hospitals are much more flexible than they used to be so talk to the ward staff if their official hours are difficult for your visitors. It should be quite easy to arrange for them to come in at other times.

You will be very tired and sleepy in the few hours after your operation and while a short visit may be welcome in the evening after a morning operation, you will probably prefer to be left in peace until the next day after an afternoon operation. Your family can ring the ward to ask how you are getting on; it is natural for them to want to know that all is well but they do not have to disturb you to find out. It is a help to the nurses if you can arrange for one person to telephone the hospital and pass the news on to the rest of the family – especially if it is a large family!

Visitors are great for raising morale, but you will certainly find it tiring to talk to a lot of them, or to talk to them for very long. Two at a time is a sensible limit and the staff, who are trying to look after you, will want to be strict about this. It is also a good idea, if there are a lot of people wanting to visit you, if someone at home can coordinate them so that they do not all come on the same day or at the same time. Children and grandchildren are usually welcome in small doses: check with the nurses.

If you are in long enough, your friends can write or send cards to you. Tell them the name of the ward; they should put this, as well as your name, and the address of the hospital on the envelope.

Eating, drinking and drugs

It is very important to starve for about 12 hours before a planned operation to minimize the chance of vomiting and possibly choking under the anaesthetic. For a morning operation, this means that you must not eat or drink anything after midnight. For an afternoon operation, you may be allowed a small early breakfast; the hospital will tell you how small and how early. If you are going into hospital on the day of operation, you have to take responsibility for your own fasting. It is surprisingly easy to forget that you are supposed to be starving and eat breakfast by mistake, out of habit. Stick a large note to yourself on the table, or on the kettle! It really is essential to remember, as the anaesthetist may feel unable to anaesthetize you if you have eaten and your operation would have to be postponed.

If you have a problem with fasting, for example, if you have diabetes, discuss it with the ward or with your own doctor. It may mean going into hospital the day before the operation in order to starve with medical supervision, possibly using an intravenous drip to keep your blood sugar level steady.

You can take your regular medicines by mouth, with a small mouthful of water if you need it, during the fasting period. Ask your doctor for advice if the instructions for your tablets say that they should only be taken with meals or with plenty of water. Make sure that the consultant knows about all the medicines you normally take, and continue taking them unless a doctor tells you to stop. There are just a few which should be stopped before an operation, and quite a few more which the anaesthetist will want to know about as they may affect your body's responses under the anaesthetic.

General points

Special diets

Any hospital of reasonable size can cope with a special diet whether it is for medical or religious reasons, in fact it will have a special diet kitchen. There is no need even to warn them in advance, although you can if you are anxious about it, for instance if you feel that it is a particularly unusual or strict diet. Otherwise just tell the ward staff when you arrive. You do not have to be a vegetarian at home to ask for a vegetarian diet in hospital and you may want to do this if you have strict religious requirements about meat and are not wholly confident about the hospital meeting them. Hospital food has improved over the years, and you should get some choice at each meal.

Smoking

Smoking will not be allowed on the ward. It may not be allowed inside the hospital buildings at all, but more likely there will be one room reasonably close to the ward set aside for smoking. You probably will not feel like smoking immediately after the anaesthetic anyway, so this break from your routine could be a good chance for you to stop smoking altogether.

Arrival

The letter you received should tell you where to go when you first arrive at the hospital – whether it is direct to the ward or to a central admissions office to fill in a general admissions form first. It is a good idea for your partner or a friend to come to the hospital and on to the ward with you. It is moral support for you, as you are bound to be a bit anxious even if you do not realize it, and it is reassuring for them to meet the ward staff and see where to come to visit you. They can also take away your bag when you have unpacked which helps to cut down the clutter around your bed.

When you do arrive at the ward, a nurse will show you to your bed, show you where the toilets are and probably suggest that you change into pyjamas or a hospital gown straight away as you will be examined by various medical staff in the next few hours.

Before the operation

Questions

Once you are settled in your bed, a succession of medical and nursing staff will come and ask you questions. You may feel quite irritated with answering the same quesions over and over again, and feel that you told all this to the consultant in the outpatients' department, and wonder why on earth they cannot read your notes to find out the answers. Don't they talk to each other, for goodness' sake?

Well, yes, they do, and they do read your notes, but actually it is a safeguard for you if they ask you again themselves. It gives you a chance to remember details you may have forgotten to tell the first doctor, and it means that several minds have considered the possibilities and checked that the facts fit together. This is better than relying on the first doctor to ask everything, think of everything and communicate everything accurately. With several doctors involved in your care, it is important to guard against small mistakes growing in transit in a grown-up version of Chinese whispers. Also, the various doctors and nurses each have their own particular slant on things, and although they may seem to be asking the same questions, they are listening for different aspects of the reply and will follow it up in different ways.

Be patient. Try to tell them everything they ask, as well as everything they do not ask but which you think could possibly be significant – such as being allergic to penicillin, for instance. In all fairness, they should also be prepared to answer all the questions you want to ask them. Many doctors are very helpful with your questions: others intend to be helpful but have an amazing knack of saying 'Is there anything you would like to ask?' in such a way that you automatically say 'No' despite your desire for several more pieces of information. Writing the questions down beforehand is a great help here.

The nurses

The nurses will probably deal with a lot of practical questions. They will make a note of any jewellery you have with you and take valuable items away for safekeeping. They will ask about any medicines you take, and probably take these away too so that they can keep a complete record of all the drugs you take while you are under their care. They will be interested in your overall wellbeing and any particular help you may need.

The nurses are the people to talk to if you are worried about any general problems, for example if you live alone and wonder how you are going to manage when you go home. They have contacts with the hospital social worker, district nurses and other people who are able to help.

The anaesthetist

The anaesthetist is the one who will monitor your heart beat and other vital functions while you are under anaesthetic, the one who, more than any of the others, has the responsibility of keeping you alive.

He or she will be particularly interested in your blood system, your breathing system and any conditions which affect your general health. Tell him, for instance, if you have a pacemaker, bronchitis, high blood pressure, haemophilia or diabetes. He will also be interested in your mouth and throat, particularly for a general anaesthetic when he may have to put a tube down your throat, so he will ask about false or capped teeth which could come loose and he will want to see how easily you can tip your head back. Finally, he will ask about your reactions to anaesthetics and other drugs you have had in the past, and whether any of your close relatives have had problems with anaesthetics, and he will check that you have had nothing to eat or drink.

Sometimes you will be offered a choice of anaesthetic, and usually there is a question of whether to use any tranquillizers or sedatives before the operation. This is discussed on page 91, and the anaesthetist will discuss it with you if you want him to.

The surgeon

By 'surgeon' I mean the consultant and everyone in his or her team. The surgeon who actually does the operation may not be the consultant, and may not be the same person who talks to you beforehand in the ward. If you want to know exactly who will be doing the surgery, just ask.

The surgeon is interested in your general health too, like the anaesthetist, and especially in your blood system as he has to avoid the two opposite complications of excessive bleeding (haemorrhage) and undue clotting (thrombosis). As well as that, he has to concentrate on the detail of your problem and how to approach it. He will probably ask about your urinary symptoms again, and re-read the results of any flow tests, urodynamic tests and ultrasound or x-ray investigations which have been done previously. He may need to repeat the rectal examination, and with the usual plan – approaching the prostate by way of the penis – he will have to examine your penis too.

There are a few particular points which you should mention to everyone in the surgical team if they do not ask about them. Tell them if your foreskin is tight and will not draw back easily. This will make the usual operation impossible unless you have a circumcision. Circumcision can easily be combined with prostatectomy, and may be advisable in any case, but you and the surgeon need to discuss it beforehand. It is also a good idea to tell him of any other minor genital oddities and swellings such as hydrocoeles or cysts which you may have. These do not interfere with the operation, but they can easily be corrected or investigated at the same time.

Make certain that the surgeon knows if you have ever had a fracture of the pelvis or any other injury to your bladder or penis, or any operation in the pelvic area. Earlier damage to parts of the system may already have used up any margin for error, so he must take extra care during the operation.

Remind him if you have haemophilia or any other bleeding or clotting disorder, and tell him about your pacemaker too. He may have to adjust the way he uses the electrical current in his surgical equipment to avoid interfering with it.

Other staff

Physiotherapists, porters, cleaners, social workers, spiritual counsellors, tea-trolley operatives and volunteers selling newspapers may all stop by for a chat at some time. It's the tea ladies who tend to ask the most pertinent questions!

Further investigations

A nurse will take your temperature, pulse and blood pressure soon after you arrive. These checks are routine on the ward and will be repeated at intervals over the next several days.

You should be weighed, and at some time a nurse will give you a clean bottle and ask you to provide a specimen of urine (in private, of course, unless you have great difficulty in manipulating the bottle in which case someone would help). The specimen should be taken in midstream, not right at the beginning or end. It will be sent to the lab, chiefly to be tested for signs of infection so that you can be given antibiotics straight away if necessary. This is important as the operation will leave a raw area very close to your bladder and it is all too easy for bacteria from the urine to invade your bloodstream and make you extremely ill. Even if you normally avoid antibiotics, you should accept them in this situation. The urine specimen also gives information on how well your kidneys are working.

A blood sample will be taken so that it can be cross-matched in case you need to be given blood, and for routine tests which will pick up problems like anaemia or poor kidney function.

An ECG (electrocardiogram) is usually done to check that your heart is working well and to rule out the possibility that you have had a minor heart attack in the recent past, which can happen without your being aware of it. This would be a reason to postpone your operation. The ECG is a simple test with three rubber pads on your chest and arms connected to a machine which traces out the pattern of the heart's activity on paper.

Chest x-rays are often ordered for older patients, especially if you have a history of difficulties with your breathing.

Choice of anaesthetic and premedication

Premedication is a sedative or tranquillizer given as a tablet an hour or so before the operation. It is not really necessary unless you are anxious and on the whole it is better to avoid taking drugs you do not need. The anaesthetist can discuss this with you and you can decide together whether you should have any premedication or not.

The basic choice over anaesthetic is whether to use a general anaesthetic or a spinal anaesthetic. Sometimes the medical situation makes one an obviously better choice than the other, and the anaesthetist will explain this if it applies to you. At other times, there is more room to take account of your preferences.

With a general anaesthetic, you will be unconscious throughout the operation, feel nothing and remember nothing about it. The anaesthetist will put you to sleep with an injection, usually in the back of your hand, and keep you anaesthetized during the operation with a gas. Other drugs are also given during the operation, and to reverse the action of the anaesthetic at the end. You are not likely to be given a muscle relaxant during the usual (transurethral) operation and so you will breathe naturally while you are asleep. For an operation going through a cut in the abdomen, it would be usual to give a muscle relaxant and have a machine look after your breathing.

A spinal anaesthetic makes you completely numb and paralysed from the waist down, but leaves you wide awake from the waist up. To give it, the anaesthetist will ask you to curl up on your side and will give you a small injection of local anaesthetic in the skin near your lower spine. Then he can guide a fine needle into the space containing the fluid around your spinal cord and inject the spinal anaesthetic through that. It is mildly disconcerting to be half paralysed, but you will not feel anything, nor will you see anything much during the operation as surgical drapes are put up to hide your lower half. All you can see of the surgeons is their hats. The operation usually lasts around an hour and you can spend the time chatting to a nurse or the anaesthetist.

If the anaesthetist recommends a spinal anaesthetic but you do not want to know anything about what happens in the operating theatre, a third possibility is a spinal combined with a sedative. This feels very much like a general anaesthetic as the anaesthetist will give the drug through the needle in the back of your hand and you will not remember anything after that. You may spend the time of the operation having perfectly lucid conversations but when you come to in the recovery room it will seem as if you have just woken up.

Consent form

No procedures can be done without your informed consent, and that goes for anaesthetic procedures as well as surgical procedures. Before the operation, one of the doctors will bring a consent form. This will ask for your consent to the operation, the anaesthetic, and probably also 'any additional or alternative procedures that may be found necessary'. You have three choices over what to do. You can sign it as it stands, you can negotiate changes and then sign it, or you can refuse to sign at all. The third choice is drastic as it means leaving hospital without your operation. The first choice is fine, if you are really happy with what the form says. If you are not entirely happy with it, if it strikes you as unacceptably open-ended, or unduly vague, use the second option – negotiate.

First of all, ask for all the information you need. What 'additional' or 'alternative' procedures do they have in mind, exactly? One possibility they may want to cover is needing to use an open operation, with a wound in your abdomen, instead of the planned operation via the penis. Decide whether you would be willing to accept these alternatives or additions, then change the words on the form until it says something that you and the doctor can both agree with. You can cross out a general permission, and write in permission for particular variations which you would accept. You can write in specific vetos on treatments which you will not accept. You are in charge of your own body, and you are the only one who knows what is most important to you. Do listen to the doctor's advice, though, and remember that you are both on the same side, both wanting to solve your prostate problem in the safest, most effective way possible.

Second, make sure that you understand the form fully and agree with what it says before you sign it. The doctor will sign it too to confirm that he has explained the operation to you.

If you know that you will have questions to ask, ask them in good time rather than waiting for the consent form which may only arrive very shortly before the operation.

Shaving and enemas

Enemas are not normally used before prostatectomy.

Shaving may be required; it depends on the surgeon and the type of operation. If you would prefer to shave yourself, there should be no objection. Find out from the ward staff whether it is necessary and what area to cover – usually from your belly button to about an inch into the pubic hair.

Immediate pre-operative procedures

You will have a bath or a shower shortly before the operation, or at home if you are coming into hospital on the day. Afterwards, you dress in a hospital gown which opens at the back; wear nothing underneath, not even your underpants. You may also be given some white stockings to wear, which are to help prevent blood pooling in the veins of your legs where it may cause problems by clotting.

If you are taking a premedication you will be given this an hour or two before the operation. The nurses will put name bands on both your wrists, check for jewellery and cover any rings with sticky tape – partly to make sure that they do not fall off and partly to avoid burns from the electrical equipment used in the operating theatre. You should take out any contact lenses or false teeth.

A porter will come for you with a trolley like a high narrow bed on wheels, with bars along the sides to make sure you do not fall off. A nurse from the ward will walk with you as the porter wheels you to the anaesthetic room next to the operating theatre, and will stay either until you are asleep or until you are well settled in theatre.

The operation

Cystoscopy

Cystoscopy – looking at the urethra and bladder with a very fine telescope – is a natural part of the operation and will always be done unless the plan is to approach through a cut, and cystoscopy has been done previously. Cystoscopy allows the surgeon to check that the urethra is wide enough to take the instruments and the catheter, and to look for any other signs of disease.

If, rarely, the urethra is too narrow the surgeon may do a very small operation to widen it, or he may bypass the narrow section by taking a shortcut into the urethra through your perineum, just behind the scrotum.

The transurethral operation

This is by far the commonest method of prostatectomy. A narrow instrument called a resectoscope is passed up through the urethra and the prostate is cut away from the inside in thin slices.

The cutting is done with a wire heated by a high frequency electric current, sometimes called a diathermy knife, and the slices of tissue are washed away by a constant flow of irrigating fluid. The fluid is a mixture of water and glycine. Salty water would suit the body better but it conducts electricity and makes the electrical cutting impossible.

The same instrument includes a viewing system so that the surgeon can see what he is doing (!) and a lower power setting which allows for sealing off small blood vessels to reduce bleeding.

This operation is regarded as major surgery, on a par with a gall bladder or appendix operation, more major than a hernia repair. It takes between roughly half an hour and one and a half hours. Surgeons are reluctant to go on much longer as the glycine mixture can cause problems if large amounts are absorbed into the body, and the longer the operation goes on the likelier complications are. This is why very large prostate glands are better removed through an opening in the adomen.

The open operation

When the approach by the penis is unsuitable, the surgeon has to reach the prostate from the other direction by making a cut in your belly. The wound is about four inches across, near the level of the top of your pubic hair. The surgeon reaches the prostate by going down between your pubic bone in front and your bladder behind. In the end, the prostate is not actually cut out but scooped out by hand so it is removed more completely but with less detailed control than in the transurethral operation.

An open operation is altogether more major than a transurethral one.

The end of the operation

Whichever sort of operation you had, the surgeon will place a plastic tube called a catheter in your penis at the end of the operation to hold the urethra open while it heals and to drain the urine from your bladder.

If you had an open operation he may put a drain in the wound, to be removed after a day or so, and of course he will stitch it up and put a dressing over it. Occasionally a suprapubic catheter (a tube which goes into your bladder through a small hole just above the pubic bone) may be used after a particularly long or awkward operation.

After the operation

The recovery room

After the operation, you will be wheeled into a recovery room. This is close to the operating theatres and it is equipped with anaesthetic machines and resuscitation equipment for the rare occasions when something goes wrong after an operation. More importantly, the nurses there are specially trained to care for people recovering from anaesthetics and from surgery. They will be keeping a close eye on you, particularly on your blood pressure, to make sure that you are recovering normally and they will also make sure that you have whatever painkillers you need so that you are comfortable before they hand you back into the care of the ward staff.

You will stay in the recovery area (on your trolley) until you have recovered sufficiently to go back to the ward. 'Sufficiently' means that your blood pressure and pulse are stable, that you are not bleeding excessively, and that you are alert enough to answer questions coherently. If you can do that, it shows that your brain is working well enough and that you have enough control over the muscles of your mouth and throat to be able to safeguard your breathing in the usual ways, by coughing for example.

Recovery from a general anaesthetic

You may wake up from the anaesthetic in the operating theatre, or on the way from the theatre to the recovery area, or in the recovery room itself. There is no sense of time passing under general anaesthetic, and you will not remember anything from the moment you fell asleep, so it will probably take several minutes to realize quite where you are and what has just happened.

It is not unusual to feel disorientated, emotionally unsteady or sick (or all three) when you wake up. Don't worry. The staff are prepared for it.

The sickness is perhaps less unpleasant than usual (because of having starved before the operation), and the recovery room nurses will usually offer you an anti-emetic drug which is very effective in reducing the nausea. They give this by injection into the buttock, so you do not even have to sit up.

You may have weird dreams, or feel weepy, or find yourself saying things that you would not normally say or believe. It helps if you realize that this is just the effect of the anaesthetic and it will wear off in due course. You are not losing your marbles, and the staff will not be disconcerted.

The anaesthetist will already have given you some painkiller, probably an opiate like morphine, but you may still have some pain when you wake. This is because it is difficult to judge the right dose while you are asleep and it is obviously safer to underdose than overdose you. The nurses will be ready to give you more painkiller almost as soon as you wake, often along with the anti-nausea injection.

Recovery from a spinal anaesthetic

Recovery from a spinal anaesthetic is much more straightforward. You will already feel quite alert, unless you had a tranquillizing premedication or a sedative during the operation. Some of the sedatives used have the extraordinary effect of making you forget everything that happened during the operation even though you were wide awake and chatting at the time. Coming round from these is rather like waking from normal sleep; it is much less disorientating than waking from a general anaesthetic.

The spinal anaesthetic will still be working when you first start to notice what is going on around you, so you will notice that you are paralysed from the waist down. This is as it should be, and an advantage of it is that you will have no feeling in your lower half and therefore no pain.

In some hospitals you may be sent back to the ward for a cup of tea in as little as twenty minutes after a straightforward spinal anaesthetic. In others, they prefer to keep you in the recovery area for an hour or two until the anaesthetic has worn off enough to allow you to wiggle your toes. Either way, it will take several hours more before you regain full feeling and control in your legs so the staff will not want you trying to walk about just yet.

The return to the ward

As soon as you have recovered enough, a nurse from the ward will come to the recovery room and stay with you while a porter wheels you back to your own bed. The staff will lift you from the trolley onto the bed and make sure that you are still quite comfortable. It may feel strange to be so passive but it is safer this way because you will still be groggy from a general anaesthetic or legless from a spinal.

Intravenous drip

When you are settled into your own bed, a nurse will probably fit an intravenous drip of plain fluid. There will be a fine plastic tube taped in a vein on the back of your hand, attached by way of a flexible plastic tube to a bag of fluid on a stand above the bed. This is not an emergency measure and it does not mean that anything has gone wrong. It is just to keep you topped up with fluids for the next few hours until you can drink freely again, and it will usually be removed around suppertime.

Sometimes it is convenient to leave the tube in the hand even after removing the bag of fluid because then it is possible to give regular injections (of antibiotics, for example) without having to stick any more needles into you. You will hardly notice it is there unless you find that it snags on loose clothing.

Recovery from the anaesthetic, eating and drinking

You will be encouraged to drink as soon as you can after the operation, which will be within a few hours, and you will be able to eat as soon as you feel like it. That will usually be around suppertime on the day of operation, or breakfast-time the day after, depending on the sort of anaesthetic and the sort of operation you had. It tends to be sooner if you have had a spinal anaesthetic instead of a general, and if the operation went through your penis rather than making a wound in your abdomen.

You will probably be sleepy for the first day or two, especially if you had a general anaesthetic, and you may notice that your mouth feels dry and perhaps your vision is a little blurred. This is the effect of certain premedications and other drugs given along with the anaesthetic.

All the effects of the anaesthetic should be pretty well worn off after a day, certainly after two days. After that, you will still be tired but that is really more due to the stress of surgery than to any of the drugs you have had.

The catheter and bladder irrigation

Soon after the operation you will discover the plastic catheter which the surgeon inserted through your penis into your bladder. You will probably be amazed at the size of it and wonder how such a thing could possibly fit in such a place! It is almost three-eighths of an inch – about eight millimetres – in diameter, not unlike the sort of tubing used in home brewing. You can be sure that your urethra is stretchy enough to take it, though, because the surgeon checked this during the operation.

At first, the catheter will be connected, via taps, to two bags. One will be a drainage bag, collecting the urine draining from the bladder; this will be on a stand on the floor. The other will be a bag of clean salty water (irrigation fluid), on a stand above the bed. There will also be a third tap which is not attached to anything. After the catheter was inserted, water was injected through this tap to blow up a small balloon (about an inch and a half, or four centimetres, in diameter) near the tip of the catheter and prevent it from slipping out accidentally.

The salty water is used to wash out your bladder, to remove the blood and debris left by the operation. In some hospitals, the tap is left slightly open all the time so that there is a continuous slow flow of clean liquid into the bladder and a continuous flow of blood-stained fluid out. In others, the tap is kept closed most of the time and nurses come at intervals to open it, fill the bladder and empty it again. They would repeat this flushing two or three times, then leave the drainage tap open and the irrigation tap closed until the next time which would be between about 10 and 40 minutes later, depending on how much blood and detritus needs to be cleared.

The bladder washouts are not painful but you may find them uncomfortable because the bladder is filled so much more quickly than normal. However, this stage does not last very long and the bag of washout fluid is usually removed about 24 hours after the operation. Then the very large drainage bag will be changed for a smaller one on the same stand on the floor, or perhaps for a smaller bag still either strapped to your leg or hung in a pouch like a sporran.

Once the washouts stop, it is essential to drink plenty of watery drinks in order to produce plenty of urine and wash the bladder out naturally. Plenty here means far more than you are used to – three large jugs of water or squash each day, as well as whatever cups of tea and coffee are on offer.

Using the toilet

While you have the catheter in place, you do not need to use the toilet; in fact you cannot. The urine drains continuously into the drainage bag and your bladder is kept empty the whole time. Unfortunately, it may not feel empty. It may feel anything but empty. It may be quite insistent that it is full and that you simply must go to the lavatory and empty it. It is wrong, but it is very convincing!

What is happening is that your bladder is reacting to the catheter and its balloon just as it reacts to a full load of urine. It is sending (mistaken) messages to the brain saying 'bladder full' and it is contracting as if to empty itself.

Not all men suffer from these bladder contractions or bladder spasms, but many find them the most troublesome part of the whole operation. Occasionally they can be so strong that they are actually painful, but more often it is just very unpleasant to have such a strong feeling of wanting to empty your bladder and being unable to do anything about it. The reason you cannot do anything about it is because the bladder is empty already, of course, but that does not alter the feeling which is still the cringeing, leg-crossing, squirming feeling of being on the brink of wetting yourself.

Exceptionally strong bladder contractions can actually squeeze drops of urine past the catheter on the outside causing damp patches on pyjamas and sheets. The nurses will not be surprised or embarrassed or angry about this; it is just a part of the job to them – but they will be concerned on your behalf if it is bothering you, and they do have some ways of easing the problem, so do let them know if bladder spasms are giving you a hard time. They can remove some of the water from the catheter balloon so that it irritates less, and they may be able to give you tablets which help to relax the bladder muscle.

There is no doubt that bladder spasms are disconcerting, but they do have a bright side. They show that the bladder muscle is still strong and responsive. When the catheter is taken out in a couple of days' time, a strong muscle able to empty itself completely will be an asset. In the meantime, try to stay unflustered. Remember that your bladder is practically empty already because of the catheter so, whatever it feels like, you cannot wet yourself by more than a few drops and there is no point in going to a toilet.

Pain

Prostatectomy done by way of the penis is not a particularly painful operation and most men find that, if they need any painkiller at all, a mild one such as paracetamol is quite strong enough. However, if you do need something stronger it will be readily available.

An open operation, one with a wound in the abdomen, causes more pain. The wound itself will be very sore to start with, especially when you cough or laugh, and you may still be noticing it on occasions even after 6–8 weeks. There will also be a general ache all over your abdominal muscles which fades gradually over the first week or two. You will probably want stronger painkillers – but they *will* be available.

The catheter may cause discomfort whatever sort of operation you had. This too can be treated: a little blob of local anaesthetic gel deals very effectively with soreness at the tip of your penis, while anti-spasmodic drugs and adjusting the amount of fluid in the catheter balloon reduce the annoyance of bladder spasms.

If you do have pain, tell the staff. They have painkillers available, and if it signifies anything more serious, such as infection, they will be able to act on it. It is wise to ask early, before any pain becomes intense, as then it is often possible to head it off with a mild drug. Established pain is more difficult to overcome.

Bleeding

It is normal to bleed after prostatectomy, and to pass small clots and pieces of tissue with your urine. The nurses will be keeping a close eye on this, and they will do any worrying that needs to be done so there is no need for you to do any. For the first day or so, the urine will be very heavily blood-stained and look almost the colour of red wine, but after three or four days the bleeding should be much less and leave only a pink tinge in the urine. A certain amount of bleeding will continue at intervals for several weeks.

It is very important to drink a lot so as to keep washing out the blood and debris in small pieces. Otherwise large clots are more likely to form and these can block the catheter or your urethra. There are solutions to such blockages, e.g. catheters with a different shape of tip, but it is much better to avoid them.

Moving about

No one really expects you to walk about during the first few hours after the operation, but it is possible to do so even with all the paraphernalia that is strapped to you. All the bags are on stands with wheels and you just wheel them around with you. However, by the morning after the operation, you will be expected to get out of bed even if you had an open operation.

The more you can move about the better, and it is worth doing even if you find it painful or tiring. Activity is a great antidote to depression, and it is the best known way to avoid blood clots (thromboses) forming in the veins of your legs. Thrombosis is not common but it is very serious and well worth avoiding. You will also find that, in the long run, movement helps to clear any abdominal pain you have more quickly, although it hurts at the time.

Some things to watch out for

General observations by nursing staff

There is a general routine of observation by the nursing staff which involves taking your temperature, pulse and blood pressure, possibly noting your breathing, and certainly keeping an eye on the urine in your drainage bag. Immediately after the operation, they will make these checks very frequently. If your recovery is uneventful, as it usually is, the frequency soon goes down from hourly to four-hourly, and later to daily.

If you have a wound, they will check that it is healing well, watch for the slightest sign of infection in it and change the dressing as necessary.

They also keep a note of the amount you are drinking and the amount you are peeing to make sure that the two amounts tally, which shows that the system is working well. So please do not use your drinking water for your flowers.

Observations by you

There is very little that you should need to worry about after your operation, but there are a few things that you can usefully keep an eye out for, particularly things which you are more aware of than the nurses can be. Pain is the most obvious of these, and another important one is any feeling of 'flu-ishness. It is normal to feel tired after an operation, but if you feel at all achy or shaky or hot-and-cold do mention it to the nursing staff. It might be the first sign of an infection and it is important to treat infections promptly because you are so much more vulnerable than usual soon after surgery.

Tell a nurse also if you feel that you may be becoming constipated. Constipation is quite likely, considering the effect of the operation along with the change in diet and the change in activity, and it can cause pressure on the urethra which slows or blocks urine flow. Modern eatable treatments for constipation are a good deal more palatable than those you may remember from childhood! They are effective too, and you are not likely to need anything else, although a small gentle suppository would be the next step if necessary.

There are two final points to watch for while the catheter is in place. First, make sure that it remains securely strapped to your thigh. Ask a nurse to fix it if it works loose because a loose catheter rubs on your urethra and causes irritation, and it allows the balloon to bump on and possibly injure the neck of the bladder. Finally, be wary of the position of your foreskin. Keep it clean, as you always do, but make sure that it stays forward afterwards. Otherwise, with a catheter holding your penis out wider that usual, the foreskin can restrict the blood flow back from its tip and make it swell most uncomfortably. The effect is like having a too-tight elastic band round your finger, except that fingers are so much less sensitive.

Catheter removal and the first pee

The catheter is taken out between one and three days after the operation, when the bleeding has settled down. The retaining balloon is deflated and drawn back inside the tube so that the catheter can slide out smoothly. It is not usually painful, but in any case it is easy to forgive some discomfort over this because it is such an enormous relief to be free of the thing.

A popular time for catheter removal is very late in the evening. Then, with any luck, you should have a good night's sleep, wake with a full bladder and have no trouble in peeing in the morning. This works better than removing the catheter in the morning and having every nurse, doctor, porter, patient and assistant who passes your bed asking 'Have your been yet?' so that by the time you come to try peeing you are incapably paralysed with self-consciousness and anxiety.

The first pee after the operation is memorable. On the one hand, all being well, there is the delight in rediscovering the sensation of passing water freely again, almost forgotten after your long experience of slow stream. ('A real thrill' one man told me, 'It took me back about 30 years!'). On the other hand, it hurts – like passing pieces of glass or razor blades.

You must carry on drinking lots of water, and not imagine that you can reduce the pain by reducing the amount of urine you produce. It works the other way. The area where the prostate was cut away is not completely healed yet and it stings when the urine passes over it, just as a cut finger would sting if you put vinegar on it. By drinking heroically, you dilute the urine and so it stings less. The pain only lasts a few days but the pleasure, the simple under-estimated pleasure of a good pee, may stay with you for months.

At first, you will have very little control over your urination. Don't panic! It does not mean that you are going to be incontinent, or that you are always going to have to rush to reach the toilet. It will get a lot better over the first few days, and carry on improving more slowly but steadily for several months after that.

During the first day after the catheter is removed you will probably find that you need to empty your bladder extremely frequently, and extremely urgently. This is mostly because the urethra is oversensitive, having been irritated both by the operation and by the catheter itself. There may well be times when you cannot make it to the toilet or the bottle quickly enough. The staff truly do not think any the worse of you for this. They know that it is not your fault, it is just a common feature in the recovery from prostatec-tomy, and they take it as part of their everyday work. Try to be patient with yourself too.

The nurses can give you pads to save you wetting your clothes, and there will be a plentiful supply of urine bottles so that you can always have an empty one close to hand. They will probably prefer you to use bottles rather than the toilet so that they can carry on checking your fluid balance and making sure that your output matches your intake.

If you do not have a natural urge to empty your bladder reasonably often, say every hour or two since you will be drinking such a lot, keep an eye on the clock and use the toilet or bottle regularly every hour even though you do not seem to need to. Your bladder may have got so used to being overstretched before the operation that it no longer responds properly to being filled to a reasonable volume, and the muscle has been weakened by being stretched out so thinly. By emptying it regularly, you are giving it a chance to shrink back to a more normal size and regain its strength, and you are retraining it to respond to a normal degree of filling. Use any trick you can to help it to empty, for instance running the taps while you pee and choosing whatever position (standing, sitting) works best for you.

After a day or two, the pain of urination and the extreme frequency should have subsided. You may carry on having urgency and a degree of frequency for a lot longer, whether from habit or because your bladder became unstable while the outflow was obstructed or from the effect of the operation itself. Do not be surprised or unduly alarmed if you continue to have occasional accidents for a month or more. Time is the chief healer in this respect, and the next chapter tells you how to help time along.

If you cannot empty your bladder yourself, a nurse will replace the catheter, using a local anaesthetic gel, and give the bladder more time to recover before letting you have another try at natural emptying. If the bladder still cannot empty itself, you will probably go home with a catheter in place for a fortnight or so. It is rare to have any problem after this length of time as the effects of all the medications you had in hospital will have worn off and the bladder muscle will have had a good chance to get over its disturbance.

Now that you are free of the drainage system, you have to take responsibility for your urination yourself and that means that you may have the problem of night-time peeing again. You still need to drink plenty during the day to wash out the blood, keep the urine dilute and promote healing, but it will be sensible to reduce the amount you drink after about six in the evening to avoid excessive urine production during the night.

Leaving hospital

There is very little formality to leaving hospital, unless you are discharging yourself against the advice of the medical staff in which case you must sign a form to confirm that you know what you are doing and take responsibility for it. Otherwise there is not much paperwork. You will probably be given a letter to deliver to your doctor, to let him know that you have had your operation, and you may be given an appointment for a routine checkup in about six weeks' time. If not, and if you want to know, ask whether you should expect a checkup or not. Some doctors feel that they are unnecessary, others arrange the appointments later by post or telephone. If you need any other forms signed, in connection with time off work or health insurance, perhaps, it is handy to get this done before you leave.

Ask all the questions you want to before you leave hospital so that you are well equipped with information about what to expect during your recovery, and about any particular activities that you should or should not do. You can still ring the ward with queries afterwards, but it is better to ask before you go. If you are still taking antibiotics or any other medicines, make sure that you have them with you, together with clear instructions about how to use them.

Apart from papers, information and possibly medicines, you only have to remember to take away your own things, including any things which have been put away for safekeeping. The hospital safe will probably be closed after office hours and at the weekend so if you have any items stored there, ask to have them back in good time. It is best if someone can come to the hospital and go home with you. You will not really be fit to drive yourself yet, and the nurses will certainly worry if you propose to take yourself home alone by public transport. Many hospitals have links with volunteers who can help patients with their journeys so do ask for help if you need it.

8

Your Recovery at Home

Do not expect too much of yourself when you first get home. You may not have an incision or a plaster cast or any other badge of convalescence but prostatectomy is a major operation and you must give yourself time to recover. Exactly how much time depends on how fit you were before the operation, how large the gland was, whether there were any complications and a variety of other factors. For a guideline, you are likely to be off work for about six weeks if you are not yet retired, and it may be as much as three months before you feel completely well in yourself again.

Do not expect too much of your bladder either. In the first weeks your symptoms may seem no better, or even worse, than before the operation. This does not mean that the operation has been a failure. It takes a good six weeks for the cut surface inside the prostate to heal over properly and it is unrealistic to expect the system to work perfectly until this has happened. Even then, you and your bladder have to unlearn the habit of frequent urgent emptying which was forced on you by the prostate enlargement. This may take months, and it will probably be some months more before you have enough confidence in your bladder's behaviour to forget about it altogether.

After the first couple of weeks you will be feeling a good bit better, less tired and with the worst of the symptoms easing off. It may seem like a good time to go away for a change of scene, and it is often easier to rest and relax if you take yourself away from home where little jobs and worries always seem to keep cropping up. Some doctors advise you to stay in their area for the first six weeks, not because they expect anything to go wrong but because they want to make sure that, if it does, you will be looked after by the same team who already know you and your medical history. Perhaps they are being overcautious. It may well be sensible not to go far away just yet, but the chance of having a problem is small and there are hospitals all over Britain which could handle it if one arose. Discuss it, if necessary, and make your own decision.

It is quite likely that you will still be on antibiotics when you leave hospital. Pick regular, unforgettable times of day to take them, spread as evenly as possible through the twenty-four hours, and make sure that you finish the whole course. Do not fall into the trap of stopping the pills when you first feel better; that usually happens before the bacteria have been completely wiped out and leaves a small army to live, multiply and attack again another day.

Taking things easy

Unless you have had an open operation, there are no particular restrictions on what you can do in the way of physical activities – lifting, walking, gardening – but there is a restriction on how much you can do. An operation is an enormous physical stress on your body. It takes a surprisingly long time to get over, and you need extra rest, extra sleep and good food while you recuperate. If you push yourself to do too much, too soon, the result will only be that you become exhausted and miserable and achieve less in the end.

In hospital, although you may have been awake all day, you will have spent most of your time sitting or lying and doing restful things like reading or watching television. On your first day home, six hours of pottering about is plenty, say from ten in the morning until one and from four till seven in the evening. This does not sound so absurdly short if you think of it as getting up late, having a rest in the afternoon and relaxing with a book, radio or television after an early evening meal. No one can judge your general wellbeing as well as you can, so be alert to how you feel and be guided by it. It usually works well to increase your active time by half an hour a day, taking about a fortnight to work up to being up and about the whole day. If you are bursting with energy and simply cannot bear to rest, fair enough, do more sooner, but remember that you have nothing to gain and nothing to prove by pushing yourself at this stage.

Visitors can be a problem in the early days. They are welcome, but tiring. A good plan is to arrange for them to visit about half an hour before a mealtime. Half an hour is long enough for a chat, and there is no problem about them overstaying as it is natural for them to leave, both to leave you in peace for your meal and to find their own. Discourage visitors from coming in the early afternoon; you should be resting then, and they may stay for hours.

If you are looking after yourself, stick to doing what is essential at first. This includes washing, dressing, eating wholesome food and very little else. It does not include cleaning the kitchen floor, mowing the lawn or buying Christmas presents for all your grandchildren. All these things can wait, or can have been done beforehand. Your first priority now is to get well. Afterwards you can get busy.

It is sensible to avoid driving for a week or so. For as long as you are tired out from the operation, your reactions will not be what they should be.

If you had an open operation, with stitches in your belly, you will need to take things even more gently. You will be that much more tired than after the usual operation, and you have to take care of the incision as well. There may still be a dressing over the wound when you come home. If so, a district nurse will come as often as needed to change it. Betweentimes, you just need to keep it dry – so have your baths shallow. The nurse will also take the stitches out, after 7–10 days.

It takes a good six weeks for the wound to heal well, and several months more before the muscles regain their full strength. It is important to keep the full range of movement by making the muscles heal in the correct position, so do try to stand up straight, walk and do ordinary movements right from the beginning, even if it is uncomfortable. It is not movement but undue loads on the muscle which can cause injury. Avoid lifting anything heavier than a half-full kettle until the stitches are taken out, and use your arms and legs to help you wriggle to the edge of a chair before you try to get up. Increase the loads cautiously (to no more than a full kettle) in the fortnight after the stitches come out. After that, use common sense as you build up to normal activities. It is fine to work the muscle now, but stop if you suspect that you are overtaxing it.

Drinking

Drinking plenty when you come home has the same benefits it had in hospital. It wards off infection, limits bladder irritation and pain on urination, and helps to wash out scraps of scab and blood from the operated area. It also provides plenty of urine so that your bladder can begin to get used to holding a reasonable volume again, even if you have to empty it frequently. Choose whatever watery drinks you like – water, fruit juice, squash, tea, coffee, the occasional pint of beer or cider – and aim to drink six pints (twelve mugs) or more each day for the first six weeks. Spread the drinking all through the day but slow down or stop in the last three hours before bedtime.

After six weeks, you can stop drinking quite so much, although it is still healthy to drink around three pints (six mugs) a day. This obviously guards against dehydration (which is surprisingly common in older people), and it is better for your kidneys as they do not have to struggle to produce very concentrated urine. It also helps to avoid constipation which is unpleasant in itself and can cause urinary difficulties too.

Bleeding

The cut surface inside the prostate is rather like the grazes you used to get on your knees when you were a boy. At intervals afterwards, as new skin forms underneath, a bit of the scab comes away and often a little bit of blood with it. The blood and pieces of scab are passed out with the urine and you may notice them during the first six or even eight weeks.

Any bleeding should be painless. You may just notice that the urine is coloured a bright pinkish red, or you may actually see a little bright red blood at the start of your urinary stream. This is nothing to worry about. The time to seek help is if you can see large amounts of obvious deep red blood, or if there are large pieces looking like clots, or if it is painful. Phone your doctor or the ward where you had your operation without delay. Obvious chunks of debris are normal immediately after the operation but most of these should be gone within the first few days.

Return to sexual activity

You can return to sexual activity as soon as you feel up to it. Some doctors advise against sex for several weeks to avoid any possibility of disturbing clots and scabs, but it is difficult to see how the passage of semen could do any more harm than the passage of urine several times a day. The operated area is not actually in the penis but higher up, in a part of the urethra which is inside the abdomen and therefore less exposed to the hurly-burly of intercourse. Be guided by how you feel.

Remember that you will probably not ejaculate in the usual way, but you should still use some contraceptive (if appropriate) in case you do (see page 47, Chapter 5). Your urine will probably look cloudy after intercourse when the semen which went into the bladder is washed out. You may find that you bleed very slightly following sex in the first six weeks; so long as it is very slight, like the small amount of blood that you occasionally find in your urine at this time, it is nothing to worry about.

Do not worry if you do not feel interested in sex for some time after the operation. This does not mean that you have lost your libido or your potency permanently, it just means that you have a natural degree of fatigue following a major operation. Do not worry, either, if your first attempt at intercourse is less successful than you wished. This is natural, too, after a long break and since the system continues to heal and revive over many months you can expect it to be better next time.

Incidentally, if you are troubled by absent erections, whether or not they have anything to do with your prostate operation, it is worth seeing a doctor about it. There are no miracle cures but there are some very helpful treatments. Depending on the cause, you may benefit from a psychological approach, or from an implant or some other sort of physical aid, or from a drug taken by do-it-yourself injection or by being allowed to soak in through the skin from a sticking plaster.

Return to good bladder control

There is a chance of some symptoms remaining indefinitely, as explained in Chapter 5, but most often the operation is successful and recovery uneventful. However, some symptoms tend to clear up more quickly than others, and some may actually be worse in the first week or two after the operation. Chapter 6 has some tips on how to live with symptoms until they do ease.

Soon after the operation, the urethra may be painfully inflamed. The pain can make the urethral muscles contract intermittently so that the flow of urine is slow or intermittent. Another cause of poor urine flow immediately after the operation is bruising and swelling in the tissues around the urethra. This swelling can prevent the urethra opening properly, causing a slow stream of urine despite the removal of the obstructing prostate gland. The swelling can also interfere with the working of the surrounding muscles so that the urethra cannot be closed properly either, and this makes leakage of urine quite likely. All these problems are frustrating but they should be shortlived as swelling, bruising and inflammation soon get better, within about a fortnight.

Frequency and urgency may be very intense for the first week or two, while the prostate and urethra are actually inflamed, and may remain troublesome until the cut surface of the prostate is fully healed after 6–8 weeks. These difficulties can last even longer if you have a urinary tract infection, which is a good reason to have a urine sample tested for infection at a six-week check. If you do have severe frequency, the flow of urine will probably be slow simply because of the very small volumes involved on each occasion.

Curiously enough, an absence of urgency in the first few weeks can be more of a worry than its presence. If you have had a chronic retention of urine before your operation, the bladder may have become so used to holding a vast volume that it does not react when it fills to a normal volume and does not signal any need to empty. The danger is that the bladder will overfill and then it will be unable to contract effectively and empty itself completely. You need to take over the decisions until your bladder grows accustomed to the new, normal, range of filling and starts signalling its need to empty correctly for itself. Start by emptying it every hour during the day. Keep this up either until you start to feel an urge to pee, or until six weeks when you start to drink rather less. Then, so long as you feel that the bladder is emptying completely and the volume produced is not more than a pint (500 ml), you can work up gradually from one hour to three or four.

Frequency and urgency lasting beyond six weeks are most often linked with bladder instability, but that does not mean that they are incurable. About two-thirds of unstable bladders will revert to stability over a period of months once the obstruction is removed, and you can help the process along by using the bladder training described in the next section. While instability remains, you may have an odd and misleading sensation of incomplete emptying when the bladder continues to contract even though it has finished emptying. This usually resolves with time, too.

When night-time peeing is caused by prostate enlargement, it is related to daytime frequency and may well be cured at the same time, although it may remain as a habit. If it is really a result of insomnia, or because your kidneys produce a great deal of urine at night, prostatectomy will obviously make no difference.

Accidental urine loss is common in the first fortnight and not unusual in the following month, but it is unlikely to go on longer. Even if you have bladder instability causing extreme urgency, the sphincter mechanism is usually strong enough to stand up to the pressures produced.

In summary, do not start worrying unless troublesome symptoms

111

carry on beyond six weeks. Even then, the likeliest cause is bladder instability which may well improve over the following few months. You do have a good chance of losing all your symptoms in the end, or being left with only a mild degree of urgency, frequency or night-time peeing.

Bladder training

Bladder training aims to increase the volume your bladder can hold comfortably and the time you can last between trips to the toilet. It reduces frequency and urgency, and very often nocturia as well. It works because the bladder is largely under the control of the brain, although it will work autonomously if it does not get strong enough signals from the central control system. If you always empty your bladder at the first inkling that it might possibly need it, it becomes accustomed to holding only very small amounts. It starts signalling a furious need to empty, and even contracting in an attempt to empty, when it is only half-full. However, there is nothing fundamentally wrong with the muscle itself. It *can* stretch to hold a normal volume, and it *can* be retrained to signal fullness only when it is really full.

Do not rush to start bladder training in the first fortnight after your operation. At this time, urgency and frequency are largely due to the irritation of the wound. It is not very helpful or effective to fight against this and it is much more relevant to drink plenty in order to reduce the degree of irritation. Between two and six weeks after the operation, frequency and urgency usually continue to improve whether you make any special effort or not, but you could make a start on bladder training if you are keen to do so. The training program becomes really valuable after six weeks, if frequency and urgency are still a nuisance when the initial healing is complete and your urine has been checked clear of infection.

What to do

Begin by making a bladder chart (see Chapter 4, page 36). That means making a note of the time and the amount of urine every time you use the toilet, preferably for a week but at least for a whole day. Look at the chart carefully. What is the longest interval between trips to the lavatory? Then you know that you can already last that long. What is the largest volume? Then you know that you can already produce that much, even if you usually produce very much less. It is not unusual to find that the bladder will hold quite reasonable volumes while you are asleep, but insist on being emptied of tiny amounts during the day. It is a great help to know how much your bladder can actually hold, and to realize that often when it claims to be full it is, quite simply, lying to you.

Carry on writing down the time on every occasion when you empty your bladder, so that you can keep a constant check on the intervals between voidings. You can also carry on measuring the volumes but it is rather a fiddle to do every time and it is enough just to do at intervals, say one day in a week.

Now that you are starting the training proper, stop emptying your bladder every time you feel like it and every time you pass a toilet 'just in case', and gradually increase the length of time you hold on. There are two slightly different approaches to lengthening the intervals between toilet trips. You can wait for an urge to empty your bladder and then delay going for a certain time, or you can choose a fixed interval between emptyings. Both methods work, but the second one is probably easier. Decide which to do and stick to it.

For the first method, start by holding on for two minutes after you first feel an urge to empty your bladder. Increase the delay to five minutes after a couple of days and then, each day that you are successful in holding on, increase the delay by five minutes more for the following day. For the fixed interval method, start with a length of time close to the longest daytime interval on your bladder chart, probably an hour or an hour and a half. For the first day, use the toilet at those intervals whether you want to or not and refuse to go in between times. When you are successful with this, increase the scheduled interval for the next day by ten minutes and so on. Do not make any particular effort to avoid emptying your bladder during the night.

I appreciate that it is easier said than done to hold on for five minutes when you want to empty your bladder, or to last an hour and a half between one toilet visit and the next. Use some of the following tips to make it easier. Try sitting rather than standing, or at least standing still rather than moving around. Pull up tightly with your pelvic floor muscles (see page 114), cross your legs (even hold your penis, discreetly, if necessary), and take deep slow regular breaths. If you have practised breathing relaxation, this is a good time to use it as a distraction from your bladder. Otherwise, fill your mind with something else, anything else – reciting a poem, counting backwards in sevens from a thousand, listing all the underground stations in order, whatever.

Once you have got over the first intense sensation of urgency, you can move cautiously and get on with other things again. It is still important to keep your mind off your bladder so make yourself busy on some job (but not one involving the sploshing of water!), or decide to read another chapter of your book or make a phone call.

As you stick at it, you will find that you can manage longer intervals between bladder emptyings and produce larger volumes. You can realistically expect to achieve intervals of 3–4 hours and urine volumes of up to three-quarters of a pint (400 ml), even starting from one hour and three fluid ounces (100 ml).

Plan to stick to the training program for a full three months. You can overcome frequency fairly quickly, in less than four weeks with luck, but it takes longer before urgency disappears. Three months is long enough for some people, but you can expect a more substantial improvement if you keep it up for six months. Even six months does not mark the end of the road. Symptoms can continue to improve for a year or more.

Pelvic floor exercise

One reason for having accidents of urine leakage after prostate surgery is weakness in the pelvic floor muscles which support and help to close the urethra. Pelvic floor exercise aims to remedy the situation by strengthening those muscles. It is particularly useful if you find that physical stresses such as coughing make you lose urine, but it is also worthwhile if the reason for leaking is an excessively urgent need to pee. Whether or not it alters the sensation of urgency, it increases your ability to hold on until you reach the toilet.

The pelvic bones have the form of an open ring, and the pelvic floor muscles stretch across the bottom of it. Strong and tensed, they are like a tightly sprung trampoline giving good support to the internal organs, but when they are weak, they sag like a hammock and offer little support to the bladder neck and urethra.

When you tense up your pelvic floor muscles, the sphincter muscles around your urethra and anus will also tighten because the nerves which control them are closely allied to each other. Relaxing the muscles is a first step in starting to urinate, and contracting them strongly stops the flow of urine (see Figures 9 and 10).

You have probably never needed to think of your pelvic floor muscles before so you may be uncertain of how to exercise them

114

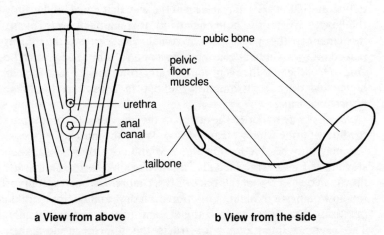

a View from above   **b View from the side**

Fig. 9 A weak, relaxed pelvic floor. **a** View from above. **b** View from the side, showing the 'sagging hammock' effect.

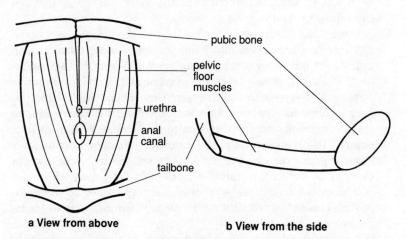

a View from above   **b View from the side**

Fig. 10 A strong, contracted pelvic floor. **a** View from above: as the muscles contract, they become shorter *and fatter*, compressing the urethra and anal canal. **b** View from the side, showing the 'supportive trampoline' effect.

deliberately. First, try tensing up in the way that you would to stop the flow of urine, or to hold back wind. If you are not aware of any movement in the muscles when you do this, try it with a finger placed on the skin between your scotum and anus. You should be able to feel the skin lift away very slightly towards the inside of your body, and the ring of muscle around your anus should become noticeably firmer.

Another way to notice the action of the muscles is to try stopping the flow of urine while you are peeing. While the muscles are weak, you may only be able to slow the flow and not stop it. If so, keep slowing it for several seconds, then relax. If there is still urine flowing, you can repeat this once or twice more. Do not try stopping the flow on more than one urination each day, and do not carry on practising once you can stop the stream quickly and completely. The exercise intentionally obstructs the flow of urine, albeit temporarily, and it would be rather silly to remove one obstruction, the prostate, only to replace it with another. The point is to notice what you do with your muscles when you stop the flow so that you can repeat the action at other times.

Once you have learnt how to work the muscles, you can do so anywhere and in any position. When you are very practised, you can even do it while doing other jobs such as washing up, but at first it is best to concentrate wholly on the exercise and to do it in whatever position allows you to feel the small movement best. Hold the muscles tense for five seconds, relax for five seconds and repeat the cycle of tensing and relaxing five times. This will take about a minute. To get good results, you should do fifteen or more minutes a day. Spread the exercise sessions to suit yourself, one minute every hour, perhaps, or three sessions of five minutes each.

It does take time for weakened muscles to regain strength, probably three to six months even with conscientious exercise, so be prepared to stick it out.

Not all urine loss is related to pelvic floor weakness, so pelvic floor exercise will not work in all cases. If your main problem is dribbling a few moments after you finish peeing, exercise may well help but you can also deal with it in the way described in Chapter 6 (see page 74). That is, pull your fingers forward from near your anus to your scrotum while pressing upwards. This squeezes the last drops of urine into the penis from where you can shake them out.

Continuing difficulties

By six weeks after the operation, most of your symptoms should have eased and it is worth mentioning any continuing problems to your doctor. In particular, if the flow of urine is still slow after six weeks it is important to find out why.

It may just be that you are emptying very small volumes very frequently so the flow never really gets a chance to get going properly, but it may be that the urethra is still blocked or that the bladder muscle has lost its strength. If either of these is true and urine is still being retained in the bladder, something needs to be done about it.

If there is still a blockage, its exact position needs to be identified and you may consider further surgery to relieve it. If the bladder muscle has been severely weakened by long overdistension, it may be necessary to use a catheter to empty the bladder completely. The catheter use might be intermittent or permanent (see Chapter 5). Some strength may return gradually when overstretching is prevented, and drugs may also help a little.

If the urine flow becomes weak again after a period of months with a strong stream, it suggests that scarring has caused a stricture in the urethra or a similar thing called a contracture in the bladder neck. The surgery needed to correct these problems is much simpler than the original prostatectomy. Later still, occasionally, the prostate can grow back to block the urine flow and make a repeat prostatectomy necessary.

You should ask advice about accidental urine loss going on for more than six weeks after the operation, too, unless it is a very small amount which really does not bother you. There are treatments which can help to solve the problem and aids which can help you to manage it with the minimum inconvenience and embarrassment. Possible treatments, depending on the cause of the incontinence, include drugs to relax the bladder, drugs to activate the sphincter muscles, electrical stimulation and exercise to strengthen the supporting muscles. As well as your doctor, or instead, you could approach your district nurse or continence adviser if the main problem is urine leakage. They are very experienced in dealing with this particular difficulty.

Frequency and urgency (and nocturia) are the likeliest annoying symptoms to persist beyond six weeks. Once infection has been ruled out, the most probable cause is bladder instability which often

117

responds well to time and bladder training. Now that the obstruction has been cleared, your doctor may also be able to help you with drug treatments to calm the bladder muscle.

Follow-up checks

Follow-up checks are usually done at six weeks. The one check which is really essential is to take a urine sample and test it for infection as this can be present without your being aware of it. There is no need to see a doctor to have this test done – all it really needs is for you to hand in a sample in a suitable bottle – but many hospitals invite you back to the outpatients' clinic to take the sample there. The advantage of this approach is that it gives you an opportunity to tell the staff how you are getting on and to discuss any possible problems with them. Some units also like to repeat the flow test to make certain that the operation has had the desired effect.

If no one has offered you a urine test by eight weeks, you could approach your doctor and explain that you would feel happier if he could confirm that you are clear of infection. With a little luck, that should be the last page in the chapter of medical care for your prostate problem. You may never need to mention it again.

Glossary

Adenoma A swelling (tumour) of glandular tissue.

ADH Antidiuretic hormone – a hormone produced in the brain which causes the kidney to take water back from the urine into the blood and therefore promotes the formation of small quantities of concentrated urine.

Alpha-blockers A group of drugs which block some of the actions of adrenalin and noradrenalin.

Antidiuretic hormone See ADH.

Baratol A brand name for *indoramin*.

Bethanecol A drug used to treat urinary retention (but not in the presence of obstruction). (Brand name: Myotonine.)

Biopsy The examination or taking of samples of tissue from a living person.

BPH Benign prostatic hyperplasia (or hypertrophy), the common non-malignant enlargement of the prostate gland.

Calculus (calculi) Stone(s), here meaning stones formed in the urinary system or prostate gland.

Catheter, urinary A tube for putting fluid into the bladder or for draining fluid out of the bladder. It may enter by way of the urethra or suprapubically, through a small cut low in the abdomen.

Contracture Permanent shortening of a muscle due to the formation of fibrous tissue.

Creatinine A nitrogen-containing chemical produced by muscles and excreted in the urine. The amount excreted gives an indication of how well the kidneys are working.

Cystometry Measurement of the pressure and volume in the bladder during filling.

Cystoscopy Visual inspection of the inside of the bladder using a very slender optical instrument (cystoscope) inserted through the urethra under anaesthetic.

Detrusor The muscle of the bladder.

DHT 5-alpha dihydrotestosterone, a substance produced from testosterone in the prostate gland.

Distigmine A drug used to treat urinary retention after operations (but not in the presence of obstruction). (Brand name: Ubretid.)

Ditropan A brand name for *oxybutynin*.

Doralese A brand name for *indoramin*.

DVT Deep vein thrombosis, a blood clot formed in a vein usually deep in the leg. It is a rare but serious complication of surgery.

Dyssynergia A disturbance in the coordination between groups of muscles, for example between the detrusor and sphincter muscles.

Dysuria Pain when peeing.

ECG Electrocardiogram, a record of the activity of the heart.

EPS Expressed prostatic secretion, fluid obtained from the prostate gland by massaging it and then collecting a small sample of urine.

Flavoxate A drug used to relax the bladder muscle and treat bladder spasms, urgency, frequency and urge incontinence. (Brand name: Urispas.)

Frequency, urinary Needing to pass urine seven or more times in the waking day.

Haematuria Blood in the urine.

Haemorrhoids Piles.

Haemospermia Blood in the semen.

Hesitancy Difficulty in starting the flow of urine.

HFEA Human Fertilization and Embryology Authority.

Histology Microscopic examination of tissues.

Hydronephrosis A balloon-like swelling in the top part of the ureter which occurs when urine cannot drain freely from the kidney to the bladder.

Hyperplasia Increased number of cells. See also BPH.

Hypertrophy Increased size, normally owing to increased function, e.g. the hypertrophy of the bladder muscle when it thickens and strengthens to overcome obstruction.

Hypovase A brand name for *prazosin*.

Idiopathic Having no apparent cause.

Incontinence Unintentional urine loss regardless of the circumstances or the amount.

Indoramin An alpha$_1$-blocking drug used to ease symptoms in benign prostatic enlargement. (Brand names: Baratol, Doralese.)

Instability, bladder or detrusor A failure of the bladder to remain relaxed while filling, instead having irrepressible contractions at inappropriate times.

IVP Intravenous pyelography, also called intravenous uography. See **IVU**.

IVU Intravenous urography, also called intravenous pyelography. An x-ray method of examining the urinary tract from the kidneys to the bladder which involves injecting a dye, opaque to x-rays, into the bloodstream.

KUB Kidneys–Ureters–Bladder, a shorthand for a simple x-ray picture of the lower abdomen showing these organs.

Micturition Urination, peeing.

MSU A sample of midstream urine, or more commonly, the tests carried out on such a sample to check for infection, for example.

Myotonine A brand name for *bethanechol*.

Neostigmine A drug used to treat urinary retention after operations (but not in the presence of obstruction). (Brand name: Prostigmin.)

Nocturia Needing to wake and empty the bladder at night.

Open Referring to prostatectomy, this means done through an incision in the skin, usually the skin of the abdomen.

Oxybutynin A drug which reduces bladder activity, used to treat urgency, frequency and urge incontinence due to bladder instability. (Brand name: Ditropan.)

Pelvic floor The large muscles which run from the pubic bone to the tail bone, supporting the abdominal organs.

Perineum The 'saddle area' between your legs, from the buttocks to the scrotum.

Prazosin An alpha$_1$-blocking drug used to ease symptoms in benign prostatic enlargement. (Brand name: Hypovase.)

Prostatectomy Removal of the prostate gland. The usual form of the operation, via the penis, should strictly be called a resection of the prostate rather than a prostatectomy because only a part of the gland is removed.

Prostigmin A brand name for *neostigmine*.

PSA Prostate specific antigen, a substance produced by the prostate which can be detected in the blood. Its level is raised in prostate cancer.

Pyelography See **IVU**.

Pyelonephritis Inflammation of the kidney and top part of the ureter.

Radical prostatectomy A form of prostatectomy used to treat cancer in which the entire prostate gland is removed along with its associated lymph glands.

Resection Surgical removal of part of an organ.

Resectoscope The tubular instrument used for transurethral resection of the prostate. It includes a viewing system, a cutting system and a device for sealing bleeding blood vessels.

Residual urine Urine remaining in the bladder at the end of urination.

Retention, acute A sudden complete inability to pass urine.

Retention, chronic A longstanding condition in which urine remains in the bladder after urination, usually applied when the volume of urine remaining is 300 ml or more.

Retrograde ejaculation The movement of semen 'backwards' into the bladder instead of 'forwards' out through the penis during orgasm.

Retropubic Behind the pubic bone. This is the commonest form of open prostatectomy. The cut is made in the abdomen just above the pubic bone and the surgeon approaches the prostate through the space behind the bone and in front of the bladder.

Sphincter A ring-shaped muscle which can close a tube.

Strangury Pain when trying to empty the bladder and being unable to do so.

Stress incontinence Incontinence caused by movement or other physical stresses such as coughing.

Stricture A narrowing of a tube, here applied to narrowings in the urethra apart from those produced by the pressure of the prostate gland.

Suprapubic Above the pubic bone. A less common form of open prostatectomy in which the surgeon approaches the prostate through a cut in the abdomen and then through the bladder.

Testosterone A hormone produced by the testes, essential for the development of maleness. See also DHT.

Thrombosis Formation of a blood clot inside a blood vessel or inside the heart during life. See also DVT.

Transurethral By way of the urethra.

TURP Transurethral resection of the prostate. The usual surgical treatment for benign enlargement of the prostate gland using a slender instrument inserted through the urethra to core out the gland from the inside.

TURS Transurethral resection syndrome. A rare but serious complication of transurethral prostatectomy caused by absorption of the fluid used to wash away the fragments of tissue.

Ubretid A brand name for *Distigmine*.

Unstable see **Instability.**

Urea A breakdown product of proteins, formed in the liver and excreted in the urine. The amount found in the blood is increased in kidney or heart failure.

Ureter The tube which carries urine from the kidney to the bladder.

Urethra The tube which carries urine from the bladder to the outside through the penis.

Urge incontinence Incontinence preceded or accompanied by an overwhelming sense of urgency.

Urgency A feeling of urgent need to pee, or of impending urination.

Urispas A brand name for *Flavoxate*.

Urodynamics A detailed investigation into the workings of the bladder and urethra by measuring the pressures in the bladder and rectum during both filling and emptying, sometimes combined with the taking of video pictures by x-ray.

Urography see **IVU**.

Vasectomy Cutting of the vas deferens (sperm duct) on both sides, resulting in infertility.

Videocystourethrography The taking of x-ray video pictures of the bladder and urethra during filling and emptying, often combined with measurement of pressures in the bladder and rectum.

References

General references

1. Fitzpatrick, J. M. and Krane, R. J. eds. (1989). *The Prostate*. Churchill Livingstone, Edinburgh.
2. Hinman, F., Jr, ed. (1983). *Benign Prostatic Hypertrophy*. Springer Verlag, New York.
3. Paulson, D. F., ed. (1989). *Prostatic Disorders*. Lea and Fabiger, Philadelphia.
4. Walsh, P. C., *et al.* eds. (1986). *Campbell's Urology* (5th edn). W. B. Saunders and Co., Philadelphia.

Chapter 1

1. Barry, M. J. (1990). Epidemiology and natural history of benign prostatic hyperplasia. Urol Clin N Am **17(3)**, 495–507.
2. Berry, S. J., *et al.* (1984). The development of human benign prostatic hyperplasia with age. J Urol, **132**, 474–9.
3. Birkhoff, J. D. (1983). Natural history of benign prostatic hypertrophy. In *Benign Prostatic Hypertrophy*, pp. 5–9. Edited by Hinman, F. Jr, Springer Verlag, New York.
4. Department of Health. (1991). *On the State of the Public Health: the Annual Report of the Chief Medical Officer of the Department of Health for the Year 1990*. London, HMSO.
5. Department of Health, *Total Numbers of Prostatectomies*. Provisional information based on the Hospital Episode System for 1988/89 operations; subject to revision in the light of additional data and ongoing analysis. Supplied by the Department, 1992.
6. Isaacs, J. T. and Coffey D. S. (1989). Etiology and disease process of benign prostatic hyperplasia. Prostate Suppl, **2**, 33–50.
7. Lytton, B., Emery, J. M., and Harvard, B. M. (1968). The incidence of benign prostatic obstruction. J Urol, **99**, 639–45.
8. McPherson, K., *et al.* (1982). Small-area variations in the use of common surgical procedures: an international comparison of New England, England and Norway. New Engl J Med, **307**, 1310–14.

9. Rotkin, I. D. (1983). Origins, distribution and risk of benign prostatic hypertrophy. In *Benign Prostatic Hypertrophy*, pp. 10–21. Edited by Hinman, F., Jr. Spinger Verlag, New York.

10. Rutkow, I. M. (1986). *Urological operations in the United States 1979–1984.* J Urol, **135**, 1206–8.

11. Steyn, M. (1988). Just old age? A study of prostatism in general practice. Family Practitioner **5(3)**, 193–5.

Chapter 2

1. Abrams, P. H., *et al.* (1979). The results of prostatectomy: a symptomatic and urodynamic analysis of 152 patients. J Urol, **121**, 640–5.

2. Akande, B. and Esho, J. O., (1989). Relationships between haemorrhoids and prostatism: results of a prospective study. Eur Urol, **16(5)**, 333–4.

3. Andersen, J. T., *et al.* (1978). Bladder function in healthy elderly males. Scand J Urol Nephrol, **12**, 123–7.

4. Britton, J. P., Dowell, A. C., and Whelan, P. (1990). Prevalence of urinary symptoms in men aged over 60. Brit J Urol **66**, 175–6.

5. Diokno, A. C., *et al.* (1987). Prevalence of urinary incontinence and other urological symptoms in the noninstitutionalized elderly. J Urol, **136**, 1022–5.

6. Frimodt-Møller, P. C., *et al.* (1984). Analysis of presenting symptoms in prostatism. J Urol, **132**, 272–6.

7. Jones, D. J. (1991). Haemospermia: a prospective study. Brit J Urol, **67(1)**, 88–90.

8. Styles, R. A., Ramsden, P. D., and Neal, D. E. (1991). The outcome of prostatectomy on chronic retention of urine. J Urol, **146** 1029–33.

9. Thomas, T. M. *et al.* (1980). Prevalence of urinary incontinence. Brit Med J, **281**, 1243–5

Chapter 3

1. Abrams, P. H., Roylance, J., and Feneley, R. C. L. (1976). Excretion urography in the investigation of prostatism. Brit J Urol, **48**, 681–4.

2. Armenian, H. K., *et al.* (1974). Relation between benign

prostatic hyperplasia and cancer of the prostate: a prospective and retrospective study. *Lancet* **ii**, 115–17.

3. Department of Health (1991). *On the State of the Public Health: the Annual Report of the Chief Medical Officer of the Department of Health for the Year 1990.* London, HMSO.

4. Greenwald, P., *et al.* (1974). Cancer of the prostate among men with benign prostatic hyperplasia. J Natl Cancer Inst, **53**, 335–40.

5. Harbitz, T. G. and Haugen, O. A. (1972). Histology of the prostate in elderly men: a study in an autopsy series. Acta Pathol Microbiol Scand, **(A)80**, 756–68.

6. McNeal, J. E. (1989). Anatomy and embryology. In *The Prostate*, p. 3–9. Edited by Fitzpatrick J. M. and Krane R. J., Churchill Livingstone, Edinburgh.

7. Office of Population Censuses and Surveys (1991). *OPCS Monitor: DH2 91/2: Deaths by cause: 1990 registrations.* Government Statistical Service, London.

8. Rotkin, I. D. (1983). Origins, distribution and risk of benign prostatic hypertrophy. In *Benign Prostatic Hypertrophy* pp. 10–21. Edited by Hinman, F., Jr. Springer Verlag, New York.

9. Roy, C. R., *et al.* (1990). Incidental carcinoma of prostate: long-term follow-up. Urol, **36(3)**, 210–13.

10. Tanagho, E. D. (1986). Anatomy of the lower urinary tract. In *Campbell's Urology*, pp. 46–74. Edited by Walsh, P. C. *et al.* W. B. Saunders and Co., Philadelphia.

11. Wilson, J. D. (1980). The pathogenesis of benign prostatic hyperplasia. Am J Med, **68**, 745–56.

Chapter 4

1. Ansell, G. (1970). Adverse reactions to contrast agents. Investigative Radiology **5(6)**, 374–91.

2. de Lacey, G., Johnson, S. and Mee, D. (1988). Prostatism: how useful is routine imaging of the urinary tract? Brit Med J, **296**, 965–7.

3. Guess, H. A., *et al.* (1990). Cumulative prevalence of prostatism matches the autopsy prevalence of benign prostatic hyperplasia. Prostate **17(3)**, 241–6.

4. McLoughlin, J., *et al.* (1990). Symptoms versus flow rates versus urodynamics in the selection of patients for prostatectomy. Brit J Urol, **66**, 303–5.

Chapter 5

1. Abrams, P. H. (1983). Urodynamic results of surgery. In *Benign Prostatic Hypertrophy*, pp. 948–56. Edited by Hinman, F., Jr. Springer Verlag, New York.

2. Abrams, P. H., *et al.* (1979). The results of prostatectomy: a symptomatic and urodynamic analysis of 152 patients. J Urol, **121**, 640–5.

3. Bruskewitz, R. C., *et al.* (1986). 3-year followup of urinary symptoms after transurethral resection of the prostate. J Urol, **136**, 613–15.

4. Chapple, C. R., Milroy, E. J. G. and Rickards, D. (1990). Permanently implanted urethral stent for prostatic obstruction in the unfit patient: preliminary report. Brit J Urol, **66**, 58–65.

5. Chilton, C. P., *et al.* (1978). A critical evaluation of the results of transurethral resection of the prostate. Brit J Urol, **50**, 542–6.

6. Finkle, A. L. and Prian, D. V. (1966). Sexual potency in elderly men before and after prostatectomy. JAMA, **196**, 139–43.

7. Fitzpatrick, J. M., Gardiner, R. A. and Worth, P. H. L. (1979). The evaluation of 68 patients with postprostatectomy incontinence. Brit J Urol, **51**, 552–5.

8. Foruya, S., *et al.* (1982). Alpha-adrenergic activity and urethral pressure in prostatic zone in benign prostatic hypertrophy. J Urol, **128**, 836–9.

9. Fowler, F. J., *et al.* (1988). Symptom status and quality of life following prostatectomy. JAMA, **259(20)**, 3018–22.

10. Frimodt-Møller, P. C., *et al.* (1984). Analysis of presenting symptoms in prostatism. J Urol, **132**, 272–6.

11. Greene, L. F. (1986). Transurethral surgery. In *Campbell's Urology*, pp. 2815–45. Edited by Walsh, P. C. *et al.*, W. B. Saunders and Co., Philadelphia.

12. Hauri, D. (1982). Life after prostatectomy. Urology International **37**, 271–6

13. Holtgrewe, H. L. and Valk W. L. (1962). Factors influencing the mortality and morbidity of transurethral prostatectomy: a study of 2015 cases. J Urol, **87**, 450–9.

14. Kadow, C., Feneley, R. C. L. and Abrams, P. H. (1988). Prostatectomy or conservative management in the treatment of benign prostatic hypertrophy? Brit J Urol, **61**, 432–4

15. Kirby, R. S., *et al.* (1987). Prazosin in the treatment of prostatic

obstruction: a placebo-controlled study. Brit J Urol, **60**, 136–42.

16. Lapides, J., *et al.* (1976). Further observations on self-catheterisation. J Urol, **116**, 169–71.

17. Libman, E. and Fichten, C. S. (1987). Prostatectomy and sexual function. Urol, **29**, 467–78.

18. Malone, P. R., *et al.* (1988). Prostatectomy: Patients' perception and long-term follow-up. Brit J Urol, **61**, 234–8.

19. McLoughlin, J., *et al.* (1990). The use of prostatic stents in patients with urinary retention who are unfit for surgery: an interim report. Brit J Urol, **66**, 66–70.

20. Mebust, W. K., *et al.* (1989). Transurethral prostatectomy: immediate and postoperative complications. A cooperative study of 13 participating institutions evaluating 3885 patients. J Urol, **141**, 243–7.

21. Melchior, J., *et al.* (1974). Transurethral prostatectomy: computerized analysis of 2223 consecutive cases. J Urol, **112**, 634–42.

22. Mudd, D. G., Deans G. T. and Lee B. G., (1990). Prostatectomy in a district hospital. J R Coll Surg Ed. **35**, 365–8.

23. Neal, D. E., *et al.* (1989). Outcome of elective prostatectomy. Brit Med J **299**, 762–7.

24. Nielsen, K. T., *et al.* (1989). Symptom analysis and uroflowmetry 7 years after transurethral resection of the prostate. J Urol, **142**, 1251–3.

25. Padma-Nathan, H. and Krane, R. J. (1989). Impotence and prostate surgery. In *The Prostate*, pp. 197–206. Edited by Fitzpatrick, J. M. and Krane, R. J. Churchill Livingstone, Edinburgh.

26. Robertson, G. S. M., *et al.* (1991). Treatment of recurrent urethral strictures using clean intermittent self-catheterisation. Brit J Urol, **68**, 89–92.

27. Roos, N. P. and Ramsey, E. W. (1987). A population-based study of prostatectomy: outcomes associated with differing surgical approaches. J Urol, **137**, 1184–8.

28. Roos, N. P., *et al.* (1989). Mortality and reoperation after open and transurethral resection of the prostate for benign hyperplasia. New Engl J Med, **320**, 1120–4.

29. Rosenkilde, P., Pedersen, J. F. and Meyhoff, H. (1991). Late complications of prostakath treatment for benign prostatic hypertrophy. Brit J Urol, **68**, 387–9.

30. Stawarz, B., *et al.* (1991). A comparison of transurethral and transrectal microwave hyperthermia in poor surgical risk benign prostatic hyperplasia patients. J Urol, **146**, 353–7.
31. Styles, R. A., Ramsden, P. D. and Neal, D. E. (1991). The outcome of prostatectomy on chronic retention of urine. J Urol, **146**, 1029–33.
32. Wennberg, J. E., *et al.* (1987). Use of claims data systems to evaluate health care outcomes: mortality and reoperation following prostatectomy. JAMA, **257**, 933–6.
33. Windle, R. and Roberts, J. B. M. (1974). Ejaculatory function after prostatectomy Proc R Soc Med, **67**, 1160–2.

Chapter 6

1. Ball, A. J., Feneley, R. C. L. and Abrams, P. H. (1981). The natural history of untreated 'prostatism'. Brit J Urol, **53**, 613–16.
2. Birkhoff, J. D., *et al.* (1976). Natural history of benign prostatic hypertrophy and acute urinary retention. Urol, **7**, 48–52.
3. Isaacs, J. T. (1990). Importance of the natural history of benign prostatic hyperplasia in the evaluation of pharmacologic intervention. Prostate Suppl. **3**, 1–7.
4. Powell, P. H., Smith, P. J. B. and Feneley, R. C. L. (1980). The identification of patients at risk from acute retention. Brit J Urol, **52**, 520–2.

Chapter 7

1. Brendler, C. B. (1986). Perioperative care. In *Campbell's Urology*, pp. 2362–405. Edited by Walsh, P. C. *et al.*, W. B. Saunders and Co., Philadelphia.

Chapter 8

1. Abrams, P. H. (1983). Urodynamic results of surgery. In *Benign Prostatic Hypertrophy*, pp. 948–56. Edited by Hinman, F., Jr. Springer Verlag, New York.
2. Mayo, M. E. (1983). Evaluation and management of symptoms after prostatectomy. In *Benign Prostatic Hypertrophy*, pp. 957–70. Edited by Hinman, F., Jr. Springer Verlag, New York.
3. Mudd, D. G., Deans, G. T. and Lee, B. G. (1990). Prostatectomy in a district hospital. J. R. Coll Surg Ed, **35**, 365–8.

Index

131